It's Not Your
FAULT
YOU'VE BEEN
LIED TO

TIMELESS PRINCIPLES
THAT HAVE KEPT PEOPLE HEALTHY
FOR THOUSANDS OF YEARS

DR. RYAN GRESCHUK, DC

IT'S NOT YOUR FAULT YOU'VE BEEN LIED TO
Copyright © 2015 by Dr. Ryan Greschuk, DC

Dedication

This book is dedicated to the dreamers; to the people who want more. This book is dedicated to the frustrated yet hopeful. Keep searching. You will find what you're looking for.

This book is dedicated to my clients for their courage and commitment for a brighter future for them and their families.

This book is dedicated to my wonderful wife and daughter. For all the adventures and excitement we get to share, your love and support are the best of all.

This book is dedicated to my brother, Jason, for reminding me to be gracious with myself, get back up, and keep life an adventure.

Finally, this book is dedicated to my mom, Grace, for displaying that true strength doesn't need to roar. Often times it's the quiet ones who are the most certain and strong.

Contents

Intro
You've Been Lied To!

"Most people have no idea how good their body is designed to feel."
– Kevin Trudeau

How do you feel when you're lied to?

It feels like a betrayal, and makes you question everything else you've heard in your life, especially if it comes from a source you one trusted. Not only that, but it can make you question the decisions and choices you've made in your life, and whether they were actually the right ones. On top of that, it hurts. It steals potential. It wastes your time. It sends you down the wrong road and keeps you from arriving at the real and important destination or goal you set out for in the first place. It delays, steals from you, or stops you from realizing or experiencing the dream that motivated your actions and efforts in the past.

What does this have to do with your health?

Simple.

What the majority of people believe about their life and their health is a far cry from what's actually inside them. There is more untapped potential inside of you than you're given credit for. You feel it too. There are powerful gifts, talents, and abilities inside of you that are 100% unique. No one is like you and no one can do what you can do. There are areas of your life where you absolutely thrive.

Based on your upbringing and your natural tendencies, you can lead an incredible life, creating something legendary, building relationships and feeling completely fulfilled. On top of that, you can have an impact in this world that would be nothing short of legendary. That's not to say that you need to be in the limelight, but your skills and abilities FULLY developed and expressed would be nothing short of life-changing.

Unfortunately, that's not what you've been led to believe. If you look around, you see that most people live lives that are far less than their best. This is no accident, and it's not your fault. When you look around you, it's easy to buy into the lie that your body isn't designed to stay healthy as you get older. Pain, medication, becoming dependent on others, low energy, and many other issues are seen as the normal process of aging.

There are more and more old folks homes, independent living facilities, medications, medical procedures than ever before. It's easy to believe your body is designed to fall apart as you get older. There are fewer and fewer seniors who live independently and vibrantly to give us a target or vision of what's possible. Without enough people living a healthy life, it's easy to buy into a lie of what normal aging looks like.

That's what happened with Stephanie, a married mother of two young girls.

When Stephanie came to me, she was fed up and frustrated, although she wasn't exactly sure what to be frustrated with. She just knew she didn't like the way she felt and that she was too young to feel as tired and worn out as she was. She was struggling to meet the demands of a young family and take care of her aging mom who needed more constant attention after her stroke. She was exhausted, overweight, and taking high blood pressure medication.

Even with these demands, she kept trying to make healthy meals for her family as well as stick to her own exercise goals. However, she found herself unable to commit and stick to a regimen to keep herself healthy. She had tried 3 or 4 dieting programs with mixed results. She came to me frustrated because she knew what she had to do but she couldn't "stick with it" and had grown more and more frustrated.

Maybe you feel that way.

Maybe you feel like you're living less than your best, held back by your health, your beliefs about yourself, your confidence, or your situation. Maybe you're kicking yourself for not being where you, or someone else, think you should be. Maybe you're carrying around extra weight. Maybe you're dealing with an illness or disease. Maybe you're held back by pain or medications. Whatever the case, you're not alone, and you're not broken.

How many times have you said or heard these words?

- I feel like I'm getting old.
- I'd love to try (insert fun new opportunity) but I'll be paying for it for the next week.
- I'm too old for that!
- My (insert body part) has been hurting for a long time. It's starting to affect my (activity you love).
- You go ahead. I'll watch.
- I feel like it's too late.
- I haven't been able to do (activity you love) since my (insert body part) started acting up.
- I'm not a young (man or woman) anymore!

You're in for a treat!

The truth is most people are being lied to every day. You've been told that as you get older, your body isn't meant to be able to keep up; it's a normal part of aging. Fortunately for you, it's just not true. You're not designed to end up on medication. You're not designed to have pain. This is not a normal part of aging.

You're told that when your body inevitably gets sick or breaks down, you have access to the best medical system on the planet to bring you back to health. Unfortunately for many, the results and experiences they have with the traditional medical model falls far short of their faith and expectations.

In terms of diet, a 2010 study done by the Department of Nutrition at the University of North Carolina found that only 27% of medical schools met the 1985 guideline for 25 hours of nutrition training for their future doctors.[1] Only 25 hours over 4 years! This was the recommendation for 1985, 30 years ago.

Given the state of our health and the rapid rise in lifestyle-related disease, proper training in nutrition is even more important. This suggests that many medical doctors are simply not equipped to help you remove one of the major CAUSES of why you're sick in the first place. In fact, it's common for graduating medical doctors to rate their own understanding of nutrition as inadequate.

On top of that, the 19 hours of training they receive on average over the 4 years of medical school are concentrated in the first two years. This arguably limited education comes before they get the opportunity to see the effects of nutritional recommendations on treatment outcomes. No wonder it can become common for patients to feel dissatisfied with the lifestyle advice they receive from their medical doctor.

Not only that, but the way our medical system treats people when they are sick has become the 3rd leading cause of preventable death. According to a study done by Dr. Barbara Starfield, 225,000 people in the US die per year as a result of the medical care they received.[2] This means the system you and I have chosen to trust to keep us safe is now the third leading cause of death, behind cancer and heart disease.

Before you think that I'm pointing these facts out to demonize or shame medical doctors or medical professionals, you need to know that isn't my intention. There are fabulous doctors, nurses, and support staff who care deeply for their patients and offer the best care they know how based on the training they receive. However, if you approach health solely by looking at the body from an "outside-in" paradigm, it's inevitable to miss opportunities for improvement or the root cause of the problem.

That's what's happened with the traditional medical system. You've been sold the lie that feeling good and not having a diagnosable illness means that you're healthy. You're led to believe you don't have to be as diligent in keeping yourself healthy because your medical system will be there to bail you out if something bad happens to you.

The reality is that our medical system has the most advanced hospitals, with the most expensive and elaborate testing equipment, and the latest diagnostic gadgets. Despite all that equipment, the traditional medical system is often ill equipped to actually show you what you need to do to restore your health. They'll save your life in an emergency, but they are often not prepared to show you the practical, how-to steps to get you back to health. If you're placing your trust in the traditional medical model to bring you back to health when you're sick, you may be disappointed with the outcome.

None of this is your fault. You're busy. You have a family, bills to pay, a job, or a business to run. You may have aging parents to take care of. And you've been told to trust a system that will take care of you when your body falls on hard times and needs some help bouncing back. I get it.

You've been tricked by slick marketers who hide, twist, and disguise dangerous, harmful ingredients as nourishing meals for your family.

You've also been confused by all kinds of studies that seem to contradict each other. One second fat is good, then it's bad, then it's good again. Suddenly only certain types of fats are good and some aren't. But which ones? Who knows!

So you go through your day doing the best you can, frustrated, confused, starting to feel the aches and pains creep up and not knowing where to turn.

Then you have people scolding you at every turn, saying you just need more willpower. You need to care about your family more. You need to stop looking to other people to keep you healthy. You just need to run more.

ENOUGH!

It's time to slow down.

It's time to be gentle with yourself and take a step back. It's time to take stock of where you are and recognize that organizations, systems, and the media are often complicit in keeping you tired, overweight, in pain, taking medication, and completely confused and overwhelmed about what it takes to be healthy.

The good news is that being healthy is easier than you think.

Step one is to take a step back and be gracious with yourself. Give yourself credit for the efforts you've made up to this point. Be proud of the small victories you've had. You've done well, especially considering everything else in your life you've had to deal with.

To explore the idea of being gracious with yourself, I'll pass you off to my brother for the next section of this book. He's one of the most discerning and supportive people I've ever had the privilege of knowing. He's been such a strength for me when I've become hyper-critical of myself. He's reminded me repeatedly to be proud of the steps I've made, and to then courageously take another.

You're in great hands!

Be Gracious With Yourself

I'm going to be real with you. Are you ready to hear good news?

It's not your fault.

I don't know about you, but in the world of health today, much of the information you hear or read is given in a way that can make you feel inadequate. The information, even if presented positively, makes you feel as if you're stupid for not knowing it. Sometimes the experts presenting the information can seem so "far ahead" you feel you can't relate. Oftentimes, the information is "too much, too fast," with no step-by-step plan to follow to make it all happen.

It's like getting overloaded with information, and then what? No plan? No support?

You know being healthy is important! I think everyone can agree on that. Why then is it so tempting to avoid the topic when it comes up? Many times it's because you feel someone is going to convict you or judge you based on what you've done in the past.

Dr. Ryan is going to do the opposite, which is why this book is called "It's Not Your Fault."

Instead of attacking you, he's going to support you. Instead of keeping health mysterious, he'll make it straightforward. Instead of condemning you, he'll applaud your efforts, and then push you to keep going.

The information in this book WILL change your life. Before he presents ANY information, Dr. Ryan's first goal for you is to have you be gracious with yourself. Before you go any further, please forget your past failures. You can't move forward if you're constantly looking back at your past. Let go of past fad diets, information that steered you wrong, failed commitments, etc.

You did the best you could with what you knew and the support you had. Being healthy is a process, not a race. It is lived one day at a time, with people who would love you anyway even though you're learning and trying to un-do unhealthy habits. The right information and the right support are essential to change. Don't fault yourself if you haven't had either of those things.

The good news is that the support and information you need are contained within these pages.

Abraham Lincoln, known for being very understanding, was once let down in the American Civil War by one of his generals. Lincoln's general made a mistake that jeopardized their position on an important battlefront. Lincoln's general, weary from battle, ignored a direct order to pursue General Lee's forces and attack immediately. Because of his delay, General Lee was able to escape, which prolonged the Civil War for many years and cost many more lives.

Lincoln felt like tearing into his general and raving about his failure and inaction. After some thought, Lincoln realized he would be the exact same person the general was and would have likely made the same decisions given similar circumstances and experiences. Lincoln was basically saying that people "are who they are" and make decisions like they do based on experiences and environment. This makes sense because what you've experienced in your past will shape your beliefs, fears, and expectations about your future and ability.

You've done the best you could with the information and experiences you've encountered.

Now, Dr. Ryan will help complete the story.

With every flip of the page in this book, you are going to have access to some of the most life-changing information you're ever going to read—about how to build a healthy life, including nutrition, exercise, minimizing toxins, having the right mindset, and the role of your nervous system in building health. In this book will be SIMPLE, TIMELESS ESSENTIALS of a healthy life.

I want to stress that these principles *are* simple. They are easy to understand. And they have kept people like you living long, healthy lives for THOUSANDS of years. Despite sustained and constant efforts to make things complicated, health can be simple. More on how you've been lied to will come later…

So take it one step at a time. Dr. Ryan will guide you. He will not overwhelm you. This is just the start. He's going to lay a strong foundation. The truth is, as you sit here and read these words, you are the best you have ever been RIGHT NOW. You've accumulated the most life experiences possible as of RIGHT NOW, and are more prepared than ever before to start taking positive steps that can last a lifetime.

What kills progress is when you interpret those lessons (failures) as if they're WHO YOU ARE, not WHAT CHOICES YOU'VE MADE. Don't beat yourself up. The lesson in each situation might have been learned years ago. Don't let that failure try to tell you who you are. You are more capable now than you've ever been.

In short, I'm here to tell you that you've been doing a great job so far, regardless of where you feel you're at, because you have been doing the best you can with what you know. Again, this information can be acted on any time. It will instantly put you on the path toward a healthy life so amazing, you never dreamed it was possible. Why wait? Let's get started…

A New Perspective

Jay's awesome, isn't he?

Now, what we're going to do from here on out is put the power back in your hands. Yes, the system is set up to keep you tired, sick, in pain, taking medication, and living a life far below your potential. Yes, it's going to take effort to come back from that. But also, YES, you can do it. YES, you will be able to start creating the destiny and the kind of life you've always dreamed of, even if you feel you're over the hill and picking up speed.

The truth of the matter is, you're designed to get better with age. I'll show you what I mean.

One of the most thought-provoking ideas I've heard turned my belief about aging completely on its head. I think it will for you too.

Most people look at aging in this way:

> Initially, you're born perfect, youthful, and flawless. You have perfect skin, tons of energy, and all you do is laugh all day. You heal from injuries quickly, never seem to tire, and are happy with the simplest amusements. You have no responsibilities and get to play all day, every day. The world is simple and easy. However, each day is another crack or chip in your being, slowly aging as fatigue, illness, responsibilities, and pain inevitably creep in until eventually you succumb to the damage of life.

You may laugh at that description, but if you look around, you'll see that's how most people view their life. They begin youthful and slowly lose their ability and their sense of adventure as their body weakens and slows.

Here's another way to think about yourself:

When you're born, you are a limitless pile of potential with no ability. You can't take care of yourself, feed yourself, defend yourself, or even wipe your own bum. As you grow up, you learn skills, discover gifts and abilities, interests that add to your life. You uncover more of who you are with each day as you pursue your curiosity. As you discover more of the world and take new chances, you learn and grow to understand more about the world, the people, and the environment. You're able to experience it more fully.

You become more effective at creating new ideas and opportunities that add to the people and the world around you. You become more significant and influential, and feel fulfilled by adding value to people. With each passing year, you uncover more of who you are and can connect to the unique traits that make you so special. You enjoy your life MORE as you grow into your skills and create the life you've always dreamed of as a kid.

Sounds like a lot more fun, doesn't it?

I think so too!

What does that mean for your life?

When you think about what you want from your life, you want to feel a sense of control over it. You want to feel good and have energy. You want to have the ability to play with your kids and not sit on the sidelines. You want to see them grow up, and you want to be able to participate in their life, not just watch. You want to be able to contribute and not be a burden when you're older. If you have a career or business, you want to see it grow and excel so you can enjoy everything you work so hard for.

All these things are great. Dream about them. Strive for them. Chase them with everything you have. With that said, you'll realize that the only way you can fully experience these things you dream of is if you have your health, and a strong, capable body.

Think of all the people you see with successful careers who sacrificed their health to get there. Now they have luxury, comfort, and travel, and they're too sick or in too much pain to enjoy it. Think of all the parents you know who are too tired to play with their kids the way they'd love to because they didn't take care of themselves. Think of the people you know who are retired and are too sick or hurting to enjoy the freedom they worked their whole lives for. Think of the people who are spending their retirement money on medications or treatments that could have been avoided.

What good is it if you build a successful business or career and don't create the life or health to enjoy any of it? There are countless millionaires who would trade all their wealth for a few more good years with their loved ones. There are even more people who are making the mistake of spending too many late nights at the office away from their family and sacrificing their health. Don't be one of them.

The good news is that this doesn't have to be you. Health can be much more simple than you've been led to believe, and I'll show you how you can have it all; the family time, the fun, the kids, the career, the success, the toys, and the health to fully enjoy every second of it!

What Do You See? What Do You Want?

When you look at the health of most people over the age of 40, what do you see?

You see weight issues. You see sore joints. You see headaches. You see low energy. You see hormone imbalances. You see back problems. You see medications. You see heart attacks. You see cancer. Just because those things are common, does that mean that they're a normal part of getting older?

No way!

Science has shown that the vast majority of health problems you can face are created by the way you live.[3] That's good news because if you can make yourself sick, you can often make yourself healthy. The difference can be as simple as the right information and the right approach.

If you think your health is controlled 100% by your genes, I've got good news for you! It's not!

Yes, genes are important and set up the story, but you decide how it plays out. Think of it like this:

Your genes form the backdrop of the story of your life. They determine certain physical characteristics, and are important in determining many aspects about you. However, your lifestyle will determine whether certain genes are turned ON or OFF. It's a process called Epigenetics.[4] Epigenetics is a principle that describes the environmental factors that tell your genes how to behave. You get to determine which version of you is emphasized by which genes you turn on or turn off by your consistent thoughts, actions, and environment.

Let me show you what I mean.

There was a lot of talk a few years back about Angelina Jolie having her breasts removed because she found out she was carrying the gene associated with breast cancer. At first thought, that seems reasonable. However, what isn't widely publicized is that there are many women who have various breast cancer genes and don't get breast cancer. And there are many women who DON'T have the gene and DO have cancer![5] How can this be?

The truth is that many of your genes have an on/off switch. The determining factor in whether that switch gets flipped is the environment you create for your body.[6] You control the environment of your body by what you eat, what you watch, what you believe, what you think, how you exercise, what kinds of chemicals you expose your body to, etc. You consistently make choices that affect how the story plays out.

So if you have so much control of what kind of life you can live, how come more people don't make the choice to live healthy?

Here's why.

Health has become super-confusing and shrouded in mystery.

It takes the RIGHT information, information that's often withheld from you. Our society is set up to keep you tired, ineffective, depressed, sick, taking medication, dealing with pain, isolated, TERRIBLY busy, and stressed to the max. It's common to live like that. However, there's a MASSIVE difference between common and normal. Just because something is common, does not make it normal. The two seem so close, but are not even close to the same thing.

Since you're reading this book, you clearly believe you can improve your health and get your energy back. You're not one to accept your limitations and live a life of quiet desperation as the vitality that allows you to enjoy everything in your life is slowly diminished. Good on you! Keep going!

Here's why we need more people like you: There are too many wonderful, talented people who have had to step away from things that they loved doing. Maybe that's you. As you've felt pain and age creep through your body, you've had to give up what you love and what makes your heart really shine and come alive, what makes your eyes sparkle. You feel like you're trapped in a cage with nowhere to turn.

It's very common to feel like something is holding you back. You've got more potential energy inside you than what you're currently able to tap into.

What do most people do about it?
Unfortunately, most:

1. Accept it.
2. Follow the mainstream approach, even though they're well aware it's not giving them the results they desire. At least it's familiar and they'll have a lot of company even if they're not getting good results.
3. Try desperately to find a new product, potion, lotion, or technique that will allow them to get healthy again. Advertisers and Big Pharma are only too happy to sell you their snake oil and incomplete solutions.

If most people around you don't have the kind of health that they want, does it really make sense to copy what they're doing and think your results will be different?

Here's another approach, and it's a loving punch in the face.

Study the people who actually have what you want!

That's what this book is all about.

It's about the time-tested, proven principles that have allowed people to stay healthy for thousands of years. I'm not talking about what some 40 year old scientist in a laboratory says. I'm talking about the people who are living long, full lives, filled with energy, living independently, without pain, surrounded by family, and continuing to contribute well into their old age. Their genes are very similar to your genes, but their lifestyle is very different.[7]

Before you think that this book will be too complicated, don't worry. This book is about making it simple. We're not going to get bogged down in technicalities. Instead, we're only going to focus on 5 main areas of your health. I'm going show you the simple steps for each area that will have the biggest impact for you. The wisdom in this approach is that you don't get overloaded with information and you know exactly where to focus your efforts.

You have a limited amount of time, energy, and money, so let's make sure you're putting them into the MOST IMPORTANT areas of your health where you will see lasting changes in your body. Not only that, but you'll understand the science behind it and how marketers will try to trick you, so you won't be a victim of their slick labelling and deceptive tactics.

You've been tricked into thinking that your body can't possibly stay healthy your whole life, and that medication and surgery are necessary as you get older. The truth is your body has all the ability, parts, and intelligence it needs to stay healthy for life. What it needs from you is the right fuel, the right inputs, and the right habits, so nothing gets in its way.

The bonus is that these habits are simple. I'll show you how. Even if you've been dealing with aches and pains, or medication and illness for a long time, you'll find out how to build a body that HEALS, year after year.

My Commitment to You

Before we begin, there's something that you need to think about. Whenever you listen to someone or read anything, you need to listen twice; once for what's being said, and the second for who said it.

So who am I and why should you trust me?

I've been guiding clients to health for 9 years now and am part of a large multidisciplinary clinic with medical doctors, chiropractors, and massage therapists that sees over 900 patient visits per week. I've received extensive training in human physiology, anatomy, biochemistry, and immunology to give me a thorough understanding of the coordination and function of your body.

I was taught to consider your whole body, not to treat each part separately. On top of that, I've become an expert in helping clients design a life so that all the changes that seem so difficult to make become easy and automatic.

I was part of a group of doctors who were the wellness advisers for multiple Olympic teams. We partnered with companies like Beyond Organic to make sure our clients and patients were getting the best nutritional advice and products available.

I graduated with honors from Life Chiropractic College West near San Francisco. I received extensive training in functional neurology from the Carrick Institute. We studied the intricacies of the brain and how simple therapies and lifestyle changes can maximize your mind and protect it into old age.

Through my guidance, hundreds of clients have been able to create a lifestyle that allowed them to implement the most dependable health and wellness habits, allowing some to get off high blood pressure, high cholesterol, and diabetes medicines. It was common for my clients to lose 30, 40, or 50 pounds AND keep it off.

On top of that, I've been able to show people how to keep their body healing from pains and injuries they thought they'd have to endure for their entire life.

I am currently in private practice, teaching my clients how to easily implement the best wellness principles so they can have the best chance at staying healthy for the rest of their life. My latest projects involve condensing the guidance I give my private clients, and turning it into easily digestible worksheets, courses, and video tutorials for people the world over.

I've also been sought out by international organizations like Take Off Pounds Sensibly (TOPS) and international radio shows through The Natural News to speak to their clients and audiences.

Most important of all, anything I advise my clients to do, I do personally. I live it. After all, doesn't it make sense for your doctor to be one of the healthiest people you know?

I think so too.

In short, I have a proven track record of showing people how to cut through the clutter of information out there and build a lifestyle based on principles that will create real health in their bodies.

Now, with all that said, I must stress that this book and the bonuses do not take the place of a proper consultation and examination with a qualified health care professional. This book is not here as a replacement for proper exam, diagnosis, or treatment, and makes no guarantees. It is here for information purposes only to help guide you in developing healthy habits, and does not take the place of a properly designed treatment regimen agreed upon between you and your health care providers. This book also does not constitute the beginnings of a doctor-patient relationship between you and I, and I will not answer questions that pertain specifically to your ailments or issues unless we have had a chance to meet in person for an appropriate history and examination procedure, and will always remain within the scope of my education and license.

Use this book as a guide to help you refine your habits and introduce foods, activities, and rituals that add value and strength to your life while slowly removing those that actively harm and steal from you.

What You'll Get Out of This

In this book, you'll learn:

- The 5 pillars of lifelong health. Remove one and your health will fail.
- The master plan that has allowed people just like you to stay strong and vibrant into their old age, for thousands of years.
- The 4 most important factors to give your body the best fuel to keep it healthy for life.
- The supercharged exercises that will allow your body to burn fat for up to 36 hours AFTER you're done exercising.
- The most common sources of toxicity and how to eliminate them from your life.
- The most neglected aspect of your wellness plan that controls all health and healing in your body. (Hint: It's inside the bones of your head and back)

Are you willing to get courageous and dream about a life of vitality and excitement beyond what most people expect of themselves? Then

I'll show you how simple it can be to design a lifestyle that allows you to create the best in health so that nothing holds you back from living the life you've always dreamed of.

Once you feel the power of your body to stay healthy in spite of everything you've been told and everything you've seen, you'll be hooked. You'll love the feeling! And it will take you on a journey that will transform the destiny of not just you, but generations of people after you.

Are you ready? Let's go!

Chapter 1
A Winning Mindset

"As a man thinks in his heart, so is he."

– Proverbs 23:7

Everything begins in your mind. This is the area to master first. Nothing exists that didn't begin as a thought or belief, including how healthy your body is.

This bears repeating.

"Nothing exists that didn't begin as a thought or belief, including how healthy your body is." Your mindset will make it relatively straightforward and simple to get healthy or incredibly difficult.

Your mind is like soil. Whatever you plant in your mind will grow. That makes it either your best friend or your worst enemy, depending on how you use it. You can plant ideas in your head of all the reasons you can be healthy your whole life, or all the reasons to be sick and in pain. The question is, what have you been planting? What have you been cultivating in your mind?

Looking at the people around you, it's easy to find examples of people who are sick, in pain, depressed, low on energy, overweight, and not having anywhere near the kind of fun they want to. Is it any wonder that with influences of that nature bombarding you on a daily basis that you start to believe that what you're seeing is normal aging? How could you not?

As this idea gets more and more cemented in your mind, it forms part of your belief about yourself and what your life looks like as you get older. You can even see it in 25 and 30 year-olds who complain about sore knees and backs, and being tired all the time. Over time, you've swallowed the lie that your body just falls apart quickly. Now the best you can do is grin and bear it as you try to get through life.

Sometimes you fight back though. You wake up one morning and decide to change how you live and get your youthfulness back.

That's what happened with Stephanie. She'd been feeling pain for years but thought it was just a part of getting older. She was so busy with her job and her family that she didn't even have the time to entertain the idea that pain and low energy were something that would ever go away.

After her mom had a stroke, the responsibilities compounded and Stephanie felt even worse. Guilt crept in because she felt she wasn't doing enough for her family. She also felt guilty for not being able to stick to the daily health-building habits that had become so much more urgent after her mom's health problems reminded her of the potential consequences. She was beating herself up and not making any progress. Despite getting great advice, she was no healthier for it, and felt incredibly guilty for not following through.

Does this sound familiar?

When you decide to make that change, here's how most people go about it.

Most people try to succeed through sheer willpower. They make the decision that there are certain things about themselves they aren't happy with, and they're going to change them. To do that, they find the best information they can find, decide on some new habits or routines they're going to add to their day, and then do their best to work their plan day in and day out. Every day becomes a battle between the new decisions and the old routines. Each decision they make takes strength and focus to resist old habits.

This can work, but it's VERY exhausting. That's why the overwhelming evidence on willpower shows that it is temporary, at best. You have to be 100% focused every moment of the day to be successful, and that's not practical because you have so many other things to think about in a day. It forces you to be "ON" every moment of the day. Eventually you fail.

When you fail, it reminds you once again that you should have known that nothing would change. You swallow the lie that health and the kind of lifestyle you dream of are for some people, but not for you. That's crushing, because it takes away your hope of creating a new life and a new destiny for yourself.

Now, the willpower strategy that most people use might make sense at first, but the reality is that every action you'll ever take comes out of the desires and thoughts that you have deep down in the core of your being. They shape how you look at yourself, and what you believe is possible for you. Whatever you believe about yourself shapes what you're willing to do and how you act on a daily basis.

Do you believe that getting healthy is easy for you? Do you believe it's even possible? Do you see yourself living an energetic, independent, medication-free life as you get older? For most people, the answer is no.

(If this is making you feel heavy and defeated, remember that your mind can help you grow health as easily as it can help you grow disease. Don't worry, the good news is coming.)

Ultimately, most people are doomed to failure partly because they haven't done the mental work to change the picture they hold of themselves deep down. Just like an autopilot, your life will always come back to the picture you hold in your heart.

It's like this. If a plane is flying across the Atlantic Ocean, it has a certain destination punched into the autopilot to keep the plane on course toward that pre-determined location. The pilot can pull the stick and veer off course, but as soon as he or she lets go or has a moment of inattention, the autopilot is going to bring the plane back on course for the destination that's been programmed. Unless the pilot changes the destination programmed in the computer, the autopilot will always try to bring the plane right back to the same course, no matter how much effort the pilot uses to change it.

Yes, you can try to change your health through sheer willpower, but there's one critical missing factor that will make all the difference in the world. You have to reprogram how you see yourself in your mind. You have to see yourself differently.

CHANGING THE PICTURE YOU HOLD OF YOURSELF IS THE MOST IMPORTANT THING YOU CAN POSSIBLY DO.

If you're currently overweight, you need to see yourself as being your healthy weight. If you're not very healthy and you're taking medication, or you have low energy, you need to grow that picture in your mind of yourself having all the health and energy in the world.

Imagine it. What does health and your desired future look like? What are you doing? Feel it. Go there and make it real, because the more you feel it, the more your new identity will take root in your heart. If you're having trouble even picturing it, hang around people who have what you want. They'll paint a picture by how they live. They'll be your visual.

The reason this is so vital is because eventually you're going to have a bad day and your willpower will break down. No one is perfect, and that's ok. With a new picture in your heart, you'll be able to look at yourself and say "Yeah, I screwed up, and I'll do better tomorrow."

You'll have connected to the fact that you ARE a healthy person. You DO value your health. Even if you take a day off or have a bad day, your new identity will remind you that you ARE healthy and you will get back to the things that you need to do to keep your healthy body. You'll stay true to the new identity that you've created for yourself.

Actions always follow beliefs. If you want to believe only once you see, you can do that, but you're facing an uphill road. However, if you change how you see yourself first, all the necessary action steps will naturally flow out of your new identity.

In the beginning, this will feel like you're lying to yourself. However, as you connect to the new vision of what health means to you, it's going to be motivating for you. Then, just like an archeological dig, you're going to slowly sweep away everything that isn't you. You're going to fully realize the health, energy, gifts, and talents that are inside.

You'll reconnect to the true you, hiding underneath all of that extra weight, hiding underneath the nagging aches and pains, hiding under the limiting beliefs. You're going to connect to it more and more. This will require consistency.

All learning is based on repetition and intensity. It takes time for the neural circuits in your brain to rewire. It's called neuroplasticity; the phenomenon of your brain constantly being rewired according to the pathways you use most often. When you meditate on this new identity and focus on the things you want, those circuits in your mind will become hard-wired and imprinted.

Remember, this is the fun part. This is where you dream. I guarantee this will be one of the best parts of your day, because this is where you decide what your life will look like. It's HUGELY motivating! This is where you take charge and accept responsibility for your life, and paint beautiful pictures in your mind of what you'll get to do. You decide.

Smile, because here's where you create what you want. It's essential to choose to wake each morning with excitement and purpose, regardless of how you currently feel.

The centenarians in Okinawa are deeply connected to their "ikigai," which translates into their reason for waking up in the morning. According to Dan Buettner and his study of Blue Zones, part of their longevity and sense of fulfillment comes from knowing exactly what's important to them and why they wake up each morning. Knowing that purpose gives them amazing clarity about what their life is about, and what they believe about themselves, their role, and their worth.[7]

If this sounds like work to you, remember that you will either decide to live intentionally, or your life will drag you kicking and screaming in a direction you don't want to go. It's LESS work and MORE fun to purposely design your life. It is possible!

The trick then is to carve out time to connect to that new identity. For me, mornings work great because it's quiet and there aren't as many distractions. Having a business and a young family means there is always someone who wants my attention, and it works best for me to spend time early on working through these dreams and intentionally programming my mind than it is to try and carve out time once the chaos of the day is in full swing.

I'm also a very excitable person, and it's easy for me to get distracted. That's why mornings work best as well. Driving in my car is an especially calming and peaceful place for me. Maybe it isn't the most common place to do it, but it allows me to shut off the world and focus. I talk to myself, imagine, and create. From that alone time, I come out with unbelievable clarity about where I want to go and what I want my life to look like.

I also make it a habit of connecting to that vision every day. Life is tough and it doesn't always go the way I want it to. There are bad days where my hope fades. Those are the times when I'm glad I've done the work ahead of time to fortify in my mind what my life will look like.

Some people say going through a storm in your life builds character and strength. I disagree. The storm doesn't build anything. The storm merely tests the strength that's been built beforehand, during the calm, peaceful times. The same storm will ravage one person and leave another person relatively unscathed. The difference is the strength and habits built beforehand.

The good news is that it's never too late to start. Every positive thought planted begins to take root in your heart and grow. In the beginning it's incredibly important to nourish and protect that seed while it's taking hold. Every time you do that, the seed digs in, grows, and eventually produces a harvest. The trick is to start planting the thoughts and visions you want, and then nourish them daily.

Now it's your turn. Where do you find that your mind is most calm? What time of day works best for you? What do you need or require to help you spend that time meditating or ruminating on the kind of life you want? Make time to dream wherever you feel most comfortable. Go there. Write it down. Speak it, out loud or to yourself. Put it up in the places you frequent the most so you can be constantly reminded. Spend time and imagine the life you want. Connect to it and write it down.

There's an anecdote I heard once about the Russian Olympic Team. Throughout their training facility they put up sequential images of athletes practicing perfect form in their respective sports. This provided a constant reminder of what the athletes were shooting for and developing in their bodies, minds, and habits. Without even realizing it, they were reminding themselves of perfect form, and little subtleties and habits that made them even more successful. The right habits, thoughts, and actions were constantly being imprinted in them so that even between training sessions, their mind had been practicing and growing every minute of their day.

I recommend you do this too. Start by analyzing your day and seeing where you can put those little reminders to help you stay faithful to the commitments you've made. Design your environment and help yourself create a community where you are constantly reminded of the wisdom and tactics of the people you want to emulate. This will keep your commitments stronger and more automatic.

You're going to absolutely love this time! Make sure you can visualize the goals and life you want because the more real you make it, the easier you'll be able to connect to it, and the easier it will be to take the steps to actually get there.

It's Your Choice

A huge part of forming a winning mindset is filtering what you allow into your life. That includes what you look at, what you listen to, and what you speak. Whatever you see, hear, and speak consistently will become deep-seated beliefs that will shape your identity and your actions.

Remember, your brain is like soil. It will grow whatever you decide to plant. If you plant watermelons, it's no surprise that you end up getting watermelons. After all, that's what you planted.

In your mind, you can plant beliefs that you're healthy and you love doing the work to create the life of your dreams. Aging well isn't just for someone else; it's for you. The more you plant, the more real it gets. On the other hand, if you plant images of disease, powerlessness, medication, and arthritis, what do you think you're going to create in your life?

Choose deliberately, because you have the power to create the future as you want it. Each day, you're planting seeds, so make sure you're planting exactly what you want.

The challenge comes from the fact that most people around you are overweight, tired, unmotivated, and living a life vastly different than the one they first imagined. If you keep your focus there, you will multiply it in your life. That's why intentionally surrounding yourself with people who are bucking that trend is so important. The beautiful thing is you don't even have to find them in your area. With the explosion of online communities, you can start to forge relationships, build friends, and find mentors all over the globe, and create a community of people who embody and live the values and principles you hold (or want to hold).

Stephanie realized very quickly that filtering the influences around her was something she'd given very little thought to. Watching the news and TV shows full of accidents, dangers, and tragedies was normal to her. While she was aware of the knowledge that her surroundings shape her beliefs, she hadn't imagined how much of an effect they could have on the view she had of her life and future.

This was enormously freeing and troubling at the same time because she realized how deep-seated the influences in her life really were.

After seeing the overwhelmed look on her face, I reminded her that realizing this truth was a huge milestone in itself. Nothing changes overnight. Courage and consistent steps are all that are required for massive change. Start small and watch as the vision for your life changes. Yes, you can do it.

This is why I'm very intentional with what I allow inside my head. I choose not to watch TV. I choose not to watch horror movies and I don't dwell on what's in the news, because the majority of it is just doom and gloom. Yes I stay informed, so I can take steps to protect and prosper my family from new threats, developments, and opportunities, but I set up my life to focus on the people and things I value. By doing this consistently, I create my ideal life more and more.

Most people give very little thought to this, and it's tragic. In a sense, they're haphazardly planting a random assortment of seeds in their mind, and then they're shocked when they don't end up with the kind of fruit or results they want. It's not always easy to filter what you focus on, but the more you guard what you allow to influence you, the easier and more satisfying your life will be.

The Company You Keep

It's been said you're the average of the five people you hang out with most. This also includes your health. The way the people around you think and the way they view the world are going to shape the way you think. Plan it very carefully. Their habits ultimately are going to rub off on you.

When Stephanie heard me talk about people and influence, she was concerned I'd suggest cutting long-time friends out of her life. She was very close with her friends and felt that it was important to maintain her relationships. Here's how I described it to her:

"In my life, there are a number of people who have been great friends through the years, but I purposely limit the amount of time that I spend with them. I still value them. I still love them. However, I recognize that we don't have the same value systems. If I want to continue to move forward in areas that are important to me, then I have to limit how much they can affect me."

Take a look at the people you hang around most. Will they help you or hold you back from living the life you want? If they help you, awesome! If not, you'll want to find people who will help you grow. When I say this, know that I'm not talking about abandoning good friends. What I'm saying is that if you want to move forward, it's more difficult when you have people consistently pulling you off course. Love them, but be careful how much they influence your thinking and habits.

Find like-minded people who are living the life you want, and stick with them.

The centenarians from Okinawa are intimately connected to their "moai."[7] This is a group of close friends they have grown up with and share a common set of beliefs and values. They live similar lifestyles and have similar belief patterns. These are people the Okinawans have known for 70, 80, 90 years! The benefit of a group like a moai is that they never feel isolated or alone. They have a group to share their good fortune with, find comfort after a loss, or seek counsel regarding some unknown or uncertain aspect of their life. Think of the bonds and the stability they provide for each other. Imagine what that would do for you to stay on course with what you've decided is important for you!

One of the biggest reasons you may not have stuck with your new habits is you feel like you're all alone. It's natural. As a human being, you're designed to be social. Even surrounded by people, you can still feel like you're walking this journey alone. This will make long-term success much more difficult for you. You need people around you to celebrate your victories and help you when you're feeling low. These are your cheerleaders and your inspiration. They're your motivators to stand up when you fall.

Fortunately, with new technology, those people don't even have to be local to you. They can be all over the world. What's important is that they share the same values as you. If you're talking and sharing with like-minded people, your odds of sticking to the values that are most important to you increase exponentially.

One of Stephanie's greatest breakthroughs came when she reached out to various online communities and connected with someone she'd known and admired for years. They'd lost touch, but Stephanie could watch from a distance and draw strength from her friend that painted a picture of a vibrant, energetic life. Whether it was a new recipe, an outdoor family trip, a new product, or something else new and exciting, her friend's life seemed very different from her own.

After re-establishing the connection, Stephanie came to love the conversations she was having with her friend. These conversations were different than she was used to. They were more uplifting and empowering. Each time they interacted, Stephanie felt better about herself. She caught sight of a new vision. She noticed it added resolve within her to intentionally create the life she'd always wanted. On top of that, she felt the satisfaction of being able to return the favour and share the information she was learning with her friend. Their friendship grew quickly.

At the same time, she noticed that other relationships that fell into her old pattern of thinking started to fall away as she became aware of the differences in how the new interactions made her feel. Finally, she started to see that being around like-minded people was crucial for her long-term success.

Make this a fun activity. As you dream and imagine your new life, find people who think the same way you do. Hang around them. Learn from them. Find out their habits, the way they think, and even the products they use. You'll love the difference you feel in yourself.

Leveraging technology and social media is another powerful way to connect to like-minded people. Online communities and communication, or even old fashioned travel make it so much easier to connect to people who think the way you do. However you choose to do it, create a community where you feel supported and understood, because eventually everyone needs someone to fall back on.

Staying Faithful to Your Habits

Oh boy, habits.

There's nothing more riveting than talking about habits. They're the least sexy part of staying healthy. Why? Because they're the gradual change of behavior over time. They're the process. As humans, we love an event, but we hate a process. However, habits are the most powerful strategy you can use in any area of your life. Fad diets and quick fixes promise easy answers, but they always fall short in the end.

Your body needs what your body needs, and there's no getting around it. You can take a shortcut, but you'll always pay for it later. Couple that with the fact that you only have one life to live, and that makes for a very high price to pay. You've seen people pay that price too. It's not pretty.

Fortunately, when you couple effective habits with your new identity, sticking to the new habits becomes much easier. THAT'S where it gets exciting! When you couple daily habits with a new picture of yourself, every day is an adventure as you discover even more of the real you.

This has been one of the most important decisions that Stephanie made this year. It's also been one of the most difficult. Diligently sticking to her daily schedule was crucial because the majority of the work she had to do involved connecting to a new picture of herself. Once she did that, everything became so much easier.

What she found is the more structured she was, the more free she was. This may seem like a paradox, but when you deliberately structure time to take care of all the things that are most important to you, you find extra time that you never thought you'd have.

It's freedom through discipline.

Now Stephanie has the time to make healthy meals, exercise, read, write, grow her relationships, spend time with her family, and take in new experiences without losing the spontaneity she always enjoyed in her life.

This was not easy in the beginning. There were days when it was tough to follow through. However, her first focus was simply being faithful to what she said she would do. It created a deeper trust for herself, which allowed her to begin to believe the commitments she made. She no longer saw herself as a liar, but could trust her own word and her resolve.

Each day she tried her best and focused more on being faithful to herself than on the actual outcome. Sometimes that looked like a 5 minute workout instead of a half hour workout because she messed up earlier in the day. The important part was that she could look back and know that she did her best, and that tomorrow, she would do better. And guess what? She did. She started to believe in herself again, and celebrated little victories that grew over time.

The good news is, so can you. Be gracious with yourself and dream again. Then rise up each day, connect to that new picture of you, and be faithful with the little things. They will lead to more.

Let's come back to Stephanie.

In the beginning, she didn't understand why it was so important for her to wake up earlier (even though she was already exhausted) and spend time just thinking and imagining (even though she had so much to do). She argued and challenged me. Each time, I reminded her everything she had tried up to this point hadn't given her results that lasted, so she may as well give this a shot.

Within a few weeks, she began coming to me saying that not only was she noticing results that she wanted, but she'd been able to resist situations where she normally would have caved to the pressure. She was able to go to a family barbecue with tons of desserts, and she had only one piece of cake. What was even more amazing to her was that she didn't even feel the urge to eat more than that.

She found herself hearing a voice saying "That's not you anymore. You don't need that." It was a massive breakthrough for her. She started to believe that she had changed. From that moment, her progress accelerated. She found she believed herself even more, and trusted that she could do what she said she would. It wasn't even momentum that drove her excitement. Momentum fades. It's not dependable. Identity endures. Instead, it was a deep knowing inside of her that started to rise. It told her "You are healthy and you are strong enough."

Once she knew that, everything else came so much easier for her. The first step was to change the identity and image she held of herself in her mind.

Remember, everything happens in your mind first. All else follows from that. When you see yourself differently, you're going to guard what you let into your life. You're going to surround yourself with people who are moving in the same direction. This is the foundation that everything else is built on. Your true nature is health. The exciting part comes from walking out your true identity and watching your life transform in the process.

TO SEE EXACTLY HOW TO BUILD YOUR IDEAL DAY,
EVERY DAY, SEND ME A MESSAGE,
SCAN THE QR CODE BELOW
OR GO TO

WWW.ITSNOTYOURFAULTYOUVEBEENLIEDTO.COM/
BOOK-BONUSES

Chapter 2
Nutrition – Fuel For Your Adventure

"Let food be thy medicine and medicine be thy food."

– Hippocrates

Have you ever felt unsure and frustrated about what's good to eat and what's not? If so, you're not alone. Health and nutrition have become enormously confusing. There's conflicting science everywhere. There are new studies that contradict old ones, and everyone has a different opinion. I don't blame you one bit for feeling frustrated.

Couple that with the fact that popular recommendations on how to eat a healthy diet are often severely misguided.[8] For example, an over-emphasis on grains is proving to be the fast track to diabetes, heart disease, obesity, and inflammation.[9] With all this confusion, it's enough to make you throw your arms up in the air and say "Forget this!"

Who do you trust to tell you what you need to fuel your body? If you've felt frustrated in the past, don't worry. There are timeless principles that are proving themselves with a track record of healing, repairing, and allowing for lifelong health and energy. That's all you want; simple. Instead you get an endless array of options and experts all screaming "I'VE GOT THE ANSWER."

This was Stephanie's problem. She had spent a lot of time looking for answers online after she noticed her energy levels started going downhill. After her medical doctor diagnosed her with high blood pressure, she doubled up her efforts. She started to feel overwhelmed by all the conflicting research.

Foods she thought were healthy weren't nearly as healthy as she was told. Foods she was taught to stay away from were now fantastic to add to her family's diet. Sometimes the same food was good AND bad. Sometimes it was good but she needed to measure out how much to eat to prevent it from being bad. It was too much! She did her best, but had given up all hope of truly understanding what the best foods were.

Clearly, food is important. It's the fuel that allows you to work, heal, and grow. The good news is it doesn't have to be a mystery. No, it's not always easy with all the misinformation and slick games being played on you. However, it's always worth it.

I'll show you how simple it can be to eat like some of the healthiest people in the world. If you give your body the best food, it'll stay healthy, and you'll have the best chance to live a long, happy life. If you don't, there's always a price to pay. The rampant growth in heart disease, diabetes, cancer, Alzheimer's, chronic fatigue, inflammatory diseases, chronic pain, hormonal issues, and other lifestyle-related diseases provides strong evidence that we as a society are sicker than ever before.

Think about your life. How many people do you know who are over-weight, have had a heart attack or stroke, are battling cancer, have low energy and brain fog, diabetes, chronic pain, or issues with their hor-mones? My bet is tons!

Ultimately, it's your responsibility to know what you need and what goes into your body. The food you eat can either create life in your body or build sickness and disease. Think of yourself like a new car. Someone will buy a new car, take great care of it, and be able to enjoy it 50 years after it rolled out of the factory. Another person will destroy that car after 5 years.

The difference is largely due to the choices you make. If this frightens you, don't worry. Nutrition can be much more simple than you've been led to believe. You have a lot on your plate already, so we're going to cover the simplest changes that will have the biggest impact on your health. These changes can be done at your pace and will allow you to simplify how many things you need to manage to stay healthy.

And remember, be gracious with yourself. Start small and celebrate each victory, knowing that you're building momentum. All you have is today. You can only live one day at a time, so focus on being faithful TODAY. That's all you have.

Plus, you've already made a great first step. You're reading this book, which already indicates that you believe the right information can open new doors for you, and that it's within your power to act on it. That's a great start already!

Study the Winners

Nutrition has become incredibly complicated, but there's good news. Here's where we make it simple. Instead of looking at piles of scientific research that seems to change and contradict itself daily, let's study the people who actually have what you want. These are the people from the "Blue Zones" who live long, happy, healthy lives well into their old age.

I'm talking about people who live into their 90s and 100s, free of chronic pain, disease, and medication. Not only that, but they live in their own home. They're able to give back to younger generations and aren't a burden on their family. They have energy and can think clearly.

They can still spend time with their friends and enjoy friendships that have lasted for 70, 80, and 90 years. They've been able to hone and perfect their skills and talents for 70+ years. How good does that sound?

Fortunately, their genes are fundamentally the same as yours. What that means is, if it works for them, it can work for you too. This is great news for you because what they do is simple. And we're going to explore exactly what they do.

Whole Food, Plant-Based Diet

The healthiest, longest-lived people on Earth have a primarily plant-based diet.[7]

Yes, meat is delicious, and we've been told we need lots of it to keep our bodies strong. Yet the centenarians from the Blue Zones show us we may not need nearly the amount of meat that we think we do. The healthiest people in the world eat meat sparingly, often only a half dozen to a dozen times a month.[7] At every meal the vast majority of their plate is covered in fresh veggies. Ideally, these should be locally grown without any pesticides or herbicides. If you simply fill your plate with vegetables, you're far ahead of the game. Here's why this simple practice is so powerful.

It's all because of nutrients and micronutrients.

In our society, we get more than enough energy from our food. When you look around, you see a majority of people carrying extra weight they don't need. All that extra weight is stored energy. We clearly have enough of that. What we ARE lacking though is nutrients. The micronutrients are the vitamins and minerals that give our cells all the nutrition they need to be able to create energy, clear wastes, digest our food, heal, and reproduce more cells to replace damaged ones.

Micronutrients are like the little screws and nails that hold a house together. Sure, you may have all the 2x4s, plywood, shingles, etc. to build a house, but if you don't have the screws and nails that hold it all together, you're not going to have much of a house. It also sure won't last a long time even if you can build it.

Without those micronutrients, you're starving yourself. You're not starving for energy, but you're starving for nutrients. When you eat food that's devoid of nutrients, your body has to sift through a massive pile of empty food to find little bits of nutrients. To get a visual, think of the biggest game of "needle in a haystack" except that your body has to play it EVERY DAY. It picks out little nutrients, saying "Here's one, here's one, here's one."

Once it goes through ALL the food you eat, your body looks at the tiny pile of nutrients it's been able to gather and says "This isn't enough!" Then it signals your brain to make you hungry again because the meal you just ate wasn't enough to give your body what it needs. So you bring in even more food.

BUT don't forget about the mountain of food your body has just digested and searched through. It has to go somewhere, so it gets stored as fat, which is often hard to get rid of. This is how you can still be overweight and "starving."

By moving to a primarily plant-based diet, you'll be eating food that is nutrient-dense, meaning your body can be satisfied, without having to process excess calories. This keeps your body fully fueled, without adding to the excess weight you're carrying. Not only that, you'll be burning off the extra fat you've built up. This means that instead of the constant effort that comes with dieting, you'll naturally and automatically start to return to your healthy weight.

You'll also have energy that lasts for hours, and a mental clarity you haven't felt for a long time. The swelling and inflammation you feel in your body will start to clear and you may even notice old injuries and pains don't hurt nearly as much.

As a bonus, it's often less expensive to eat this way, so you'll have extra cash every month to take your family somewhere special or to treat yourself to something nice. The highest concentrations of centenarians often come from less affluent areas of the world, meaning you don't need to spend big money to get nutrient-dense, super-healthy foods.

You may be saying "I can't do that; I love meat!"

This was what Stephanie said after our first few sessions. She and her family love meat. They love to barbecue in the summer. But what she found was the healthier she started to eat, the less she craved it. She didn't even try to cut it out, but instead focused on ADDING healthy fruits and vegetables, beans, legumes, nuts, and seeds.

No one likes depriving themselves of something they enjoy, so focus on ADDING in healthy fruits and vegetables BEFORE SUBTRACTING meat. (This tactic of ADDING good food before SUBTRACTING also works for breaking cravings for sweets or junk food). As Stephanie added those foods, she slowly shifted to needing less meat. Once she felt her energy rise, her sleep improve, and her body start to lean out, she was hooked.

Start with ADDITION before SUBTRACTION. Add nutrient-dense, plant-based foods before you remove the unhealthy foods you're accustomed to. This will help you make the transition smoother and ultimately make you more successful in the long run.

Your Two Biggest Enemies

When it comes to your health, the long-term issues you face can often be tied to two things: **inflammation and insulin resistance**. These are two of the culprits that contribute to brain fog, fatigue, issues with regulating hormones, diabetes, heart disease, cancer, etc.[11]

1. Inflammation
First off, what is inflammation?

Inflammation is your body's response to injury. Normally it happens when you physically hurt yourself, or your body has to mount an attack against something that doesn't belong there. You experience swelling, your temperature rises, you feel drained of energy, your nose runs, your eyes water, and your immune system kicks into high gear. It's essentially a war zone, where your body is battling and rapidly patching up various areas that have been damaged.

Normally, inflammation is meant to be a short-term solution because of all the collateral damage it causes in your body, in addition to the effect it has on your growth and repair processes. Despite the damage, this is actually an intelligent response from your body because in the middle of a war zone, you're more concerned with patching up the damaged areas as fast as possible than you are with making sure everything is neat, orderly, cleaned up and working at 100%. It's pure survival mode at that point!

The way you've been eating has likely forced your body to live in this survival, crisis mode for quite some time. Foods that trigger inflammation cause collateral damage everywhere. This uses massive amounts of energy to keep up a constant battle, which can leave you constantly tired. It wears down every part of your body day in and day out.

Is it any wonder you're hurting and zapped of energy? This low-grade, constant "injury" your body is facing damages your blood vessels, leading to the buildup of plaque on the inside of your vessel walls, which causes them to narrow and plug up.[11] It damages the cartilage in your joints, leading to arthritis and pain.[11] It sensitizes your nerves, making any pain that you have in your body automatically FEEL worse. It damages your heart and all your organs.[11] It makes you feel bloated and puffy. It's just no good.

On top of that, constant low grade inflammation from having an unhealthy gut has major effects on your mental health.[11] New research shows you have more neurotransmitters in your gut than you do in your brain. Your brain relies on proper communication from your gut to form an accurate picture of your surroundings and environment so it can respond normally and appropriately.

When your gut is unhealthy from foods that lack nutrients, it becomes "leaky," allowing molecules to cross the blood/brain barrier without proper regulation and wreak havoc with your mental state. By restoring the quality of the nutrients in the foods you eat, you'll not only begin to heal your body, but your mental health can improve as well.

2. Insulin Resistance

Insulin resistance is all about sugar. We eat far too much sugar. Back in the early 1900s, the average person would eat approximately 5 pounds a year. Now, the average is 150 pounds![12] 150 POUNDS!

Now, you're likely thinking 1 of 2 things. Either you're absolutely shocked at how it's possible to eat 150 pounds of sugar in a year, or you're saying "Good thing I don't eat anywhere near that amount." Don't go congratulating yourself just yet. When we talk about sugar, you have to realize we're talking sugar AND all the sources of sugar. That includes bread, rice, pasta, potatoes, and processed foods (anything preserved or in a box), as well as fruit.[12]

You may be thinking, "Isn't fruit good for you?" Yes, but when you look at ALL the sources of sugar, it adds to the burden of sugar your body has to process on a daily basis. Many clients have found they see faster results when they focus on vegetables instead of fruits while they're getting their sugar levels back in line.

Here's what too much sugar does to your body.

Imagine a factory with a conveyor belt running down the middle and machines placed on each side. At each machine is a worker who's responsible for feeding fuel into the machines as it comes down the conveyor. Each day, approximately 3 times a day, supplies are delivered on the conveyor to keep the machines running. In a perfect world, just enough supplies are delivered to keep the machines fired up and working perfectly.

At the front of the factory is a soft-spoken man named Ivan. Ivan's job is to tell each worker at the machine to feed the machine as the recently delivered supplies move past. Normally, his job is pretty easy because the workers are happy to listen to him and keep the machines filled and running well.

Lately though, more supplies have been delivered than are necessary to run the machines. At first, this is no problem because Ivan can politely ask his workers to work a little harder to burn up all the supplies, and everything returns to normal. The machines had to work a little harder, but they can do that from time to time.

This continues to happen daily, though, and Ivan finds he has to be increasingly forceful each time to get his workers to burn up the supplies each day. They start to ignore him because they know that burning all these extra supplies is damaging the machines.

Eventually, Ivan is screaming at the workers to load all the extra supplies into the machines and the workers are completely ignoring him.

The supplies start to pile up in the factory and clog the conveyor belt. Since the supplies can't be burned, they have to be stored. In time, every single one of the factory's store rooms are filled with excess supplies. The factory is congested and stops working like the well-oiled, new factory it once was.

In this story, Ivan is your hormone insulin. Insulin is responsible for telling your cells to take in sugar for fuel. Over time, too much sugar causes the receptors on your cells to stop listening to insulin's commands. Sugar builds up in your bloodstream. This can cause a TON of terrible things in your body if it's not put somewhere.

When sugar is stored in your body, you get fat. This is a very smart thing for your body to do. You can't have excess sugar floating around your bloodstream because it leads to all kinds of nasty consequences. It can cause massive bacterial infections, nerve damage, destruction of artery walls, kidney damage, blindness, as well as inflammation EVERYWHERE in your body.[13]

Here's another fact for you. Sugar is the only fuel that cancer can use to grow. We've known this since 1931. (That's a while ago...) Dr. Otto Warburg found that:

> "All normal body cells meet their energy needs by respiration of oxygen, whereas cancer cells meet their energy needs in great part by fermentation. All normal body cells are thus obligate aerobes, whereas all cancer cells are partial anaerobes. From the standpoint of the physics and chemistry of life this difference between normal and cancer cells is so great that one can scarcely picture a greater difference. Oxygen gas, the donor of energy in plants and animals, is dethroned in the cancer cells and replaced by the energy-yielding reaction of the lowest living forms, namely the fermentation of sugar."[14]

What this means is that normal cells get their energy from oxygen (respiration). Because normal cells have to work and coordinate with other cells in your body, they require more energy. That's why their primary fuel is oxygen.

Cancer cells are damaged cells that become concerned only with their own survival. As a result, they can no longer use oxygen for fuel and instead run entirely on sugar to grow and spread.[15] Cancer cells have damaged mitochondria (engines) that can't use oxygen for energy anymore, even though oxygen provides FAR MORE energy for the cell. The cancer cells are forced to use sugar to grow. Cancer needs a constant supply of sugar to feed itself because it's fast growing, and sugar provides far less energy than oxygen would.

In fact, when oncologists try to find out exactly where cancerous tumours are growing in a patient's body, they do a PET scan.[15] This involves injecting radioactive sugar and then looking to see where that sugar concentrates in the body. Why? Because cancer will gobble up the sugar, since sugar is the only fuel cancer can use to grow. As a result, higher concentrations of this radioactive sugar highlight exactly where these cancerous tumours are present.

When you bring in more sugar than you need, you're giving cancer its preferred fuel and helping sustain its growth and expansion.[16]

Elevated blood sugar (and the inflammation that results from it) has also been attributed to the development and progression of Alzheimer's.[17] Some researchers have suggested referring to Alzheimer's as "Type 3 Diabetes." As I mentioned earlier, the inflammation created by all the extra sugar is able to cross the blood/brain barrier, ultimately destroying brain and nerve cells. If you've ever seen or known anyone with Alzheimer's, it's absolutely devastating.

In the world around you, inflammation and insulin resistance are the two biggest causes of the problems you'll face, especially as it relates to lifestyle and inflammatory diseases. Fortunately, the solution is relatively straightforward.

So What's the Solution?

Enough about the problem; what do you do about it? You've heard all the fad diets out there designed by fitness gurus and scientists. There's no shortage of new scientific breakthroughs, new pills, rare herbs, or celebrity endorsements. You're constantly bombarded with them. They may get you results, but they've all been tested for only a short time.

That's great, but wouldn't you rather trust the principles that have kept people healthy for thousands of years? You only have a certain amount of time, energy, and money, and you don't want to waste any of them.

Here's where it can be much more simple. The centenarians in the Blue Zones are living proof of what it takes to be healthy. Rather than complicate things, let's just do what they do. Doesn't that make more sense?

Perfect. I think so too.

We're going to focus on 4 simple principles. Only 4. Why only 4? Because mastering these foundational principles makes you far more likely to succeed and see results long term. Master these first and then fine tune once you've laid a strong foundation.

Here's your solution:

- Reduce/eliminate sugar (and sources of sugar)
- Increase healthy fats
- Moderate protein intake
- Remove toxins

1. Reduce sugar and sources of sugar. This is one of the MOST POWERFUL actions you can do to start rebuilding your body. We eat way too much sugar because it's EVERYWHERE. By reducing sugar and sources of sugar, you'll create a lean, strong, energized body that will stay healthy for years to come.

Sources of sugar include foods like bread, rice, pasta, potatoes, and processed foods. One of the secrets of the Blue Zones is that their sugar sources are paired with FIBER. Fiber is the indigestible part of the plant that slows how quickly your body can absorb the sugar. By slowing how fast your body can absorb sugar, you minimize how high your insulin levels spike. Ivan doesn't have to scream as loudly at his workers and they do a better job of listening and clear sugar from your bloodstream into your cells. This keeps your blood sugar levels in check and your cells healthy.

If you're concerned about how to sweeten the foods you eat without adding sugar, try **stevia or xylitol.** They aren't synthetic sweeteners like aspartame or sucralose, and won't spike your blood sugar.

2. Increase your intake of healthy fats. For the longest time you've been sold the lie that all fat is bad. This attitude is changing over time, but you may not be aware of how essential good fat is for your body.

Good fats allow your body to build hormones and absorb vitamins. Not only that, but every cell in your body has a double layer of fat that allows it to properly sense and respond to the outside environment. If they don't get the right fats, your cells are completely guessing about what to do next because they can't sense the minute-by-minute demands that come from an ever-changing environment within and around you. This is a big deal because if your cells aren't healthy and working together, they won't be able to coordinate as well to keep you healthy or to make the appropriate decisions at the right time.

Your brain and nerve cells also have a layer of fat that allow them to communicate at lightning speeds. Cut down on your intake of healthy fats and you're putting handcuffs on your brain's ability to think and control every part of your body.

Healthy fat is also essential for you to reduce inflammation that's built up in your body as well as to burn up the fat that's been stored.

What are the sources of good and bad fats?

Good fats – coconut oil, avocado oil, olive oil, butter, unpasteurized cheese, grass fed meats, wild caught Pacific fish, nuts and seeds.

Bad fats – margarine, vegetable oil, canola oil, soybean oil, safflower oil, processed foods.

3. Moderate your protein intake. Yes, you need protein to rebuild your body. No, you don't need to eat as much meat as you think. The healthiest people in the world eat meat sparingly. According to Dan Buettner's research on Blue Zones, they eat meat less than a dozen times a month on average.[7]

This is especially important for you now, because the meat you get from the grocery store or even specialty stores is often LOADED with hormones, steroids, antibiotics and all kinds of toxic chemicals. It's common today for meat to be washed down with bleach to kill off any bacteria or germs.[18] Doesn't that sound delicious?

Too much protein will also trigger your body to convert the excess protein into sugar, and you just read about the problems excess sugar will create for you. There are tons of foods like broccoli, beans, chick peas, chia seeds, or hemp seeds that will give you enough protein without overloading your body, and help you lessen the amount of meat you consume on a weekly basis.

4. Reduce toxins. There is a whole section devoted to toxicity later in this book.

I'll touch on it briefly here. Synthetic chemicals are not natural, and your body can have a difficult time processing and eliminating them. They hurt you in all kinds of nasty ways, from inflammation to cellular and DNA damage, to accumulation in your organs. If you want to live a long life, you need to stop putting them in your body. Buying organic food is a great start. However, you don't have unlimited money to spend, so I've included a guide in the bonus section to help you prioritize.

The Environmental Working Group puts out a fantastic chart every year that will help you prioritize which foods are ok to buy non-organic, and which foods are so loaded with pesticides and chemicals that it's recommended you buy them organically grown. I've brought it to you neatly packaged.

TO GET YOUR COPY OF THE EWG'S CLEAN 15/
DIRTY DOZEN SCAN THE QR CODE BELOW
OR GO TO

WWW.ITSNOTYOURFAULTYOUVEBEENLIEDTO.COM/
BOOK-BONUSES

Build a Strong Foundation

The first step in moving forward is making the decision. Once you've made a decision, you'll find the way. By focusing on a few changes, you'll be able to focus on mastering them, and enjoying the results you're seeing. Not only that, but you can be confident in knowing that these principles have been are backed up by the proven habits of longevity cultures all over the world.

If you still feel uncertain of where to start, I'll show you how to take the unhealthy recipes you love and make them completely healthy.

Once a month, I open my house to clients and guests and we have a BIG party where I make healthy recipes for them. They get to hear the ins and outs of every ingredient. At the end, they leave confident and equipped to modify any recipe so that it's only healthy food going in their mouths. It's all about making it easy on you.

In the past, we've made brownies, pasta with pesto, pancakes, chocolate cake, power bars, lasagna, and pizza. The options are only limited by your knowledge and imagination.

TO COME TO THE NEXT REAL FOOD FIESTA – SHOWING YOU HOW YOU CAN MAKE YOUR FAVOURITE RECIPES SUPER HEALTHY AND STILL ENJOY THEM, GO TO WWW.FACEBOOK.COM/ASKDRRYAN

WWW.ITSNOTYOURFAULTYOUVEBEENLIEDTO.COM/ BOOK-BONUSES

Supplements – Which Do I Need?

At this point, you may be wondering about the role supplements play in staying healthy. You may also be wondering how to sort through ALL the supplements you CAN take, so you can focus on the most important.

As always, let's start with a strong foundation.

In a perfect world, the best source of nutrients is always real food. Real food has all the vitamins, minerals, and co-factors that occur to-gether so you can absorb and digest the good stuff in the best, most natural way. The bad news is the food you eat has often been modi-fied in a way that diminishes the nutrient quality of your food. This can happen because of how depleted our soils often are, genetic modi-fication, or other alterations that have been done to the food you eat.

We have more food than ever before, but there are concerns about how nutritious that food is. If you want to stay healthy for life, food may not be enough. This makes supplements essential to give your body everything it needs to stay well. In my practice, I only focus on the few that will make the biggest impact on your health.

These will give you the strongest foundation for your health:

- **A quality multivitamin.** It's important to make sure it is COMPLETE, PURE, EASILY ABSORBED, and from HIGH QUALITY INGREDIENTS. HERE'S WHY;
www.itsnotyourfaultyouvebeenliedto.com/book-bonuses/
- **Vitamin D3.** The old recommendation of 400 IU/day is gross-ly inadequate. According to the Vitamin D Council, 5000 IU/day is the level you want to be shooting for. HERE'S WHY; www.itsnotyourfaultyouvebeenliedto.com/book-bonuses/
- **A quality omega 3** supplement from small fish, to avoid high levels of toxicity found in larger fish.

- **A glutathione booster** to keep your detox pathways and immune system strong. The trick is to get the "precursors to glutathione" because glutathione is destroyed in your stomach if you try to ingest it as a complete molecule. HERE'S WHY; www.itsnotyourfaultyouvebeenliedto.com/book-bonuses/

- **A quality collagen or protein.** Quality animal protein allows you a highly absorbable protein source with no hormones or antibiotics. This makes reducing meat even easier because your body still gets the protein it needs to rebuild and repair. A collagen supplement also helps you rebuild the entire structure of your body, including bones, joints, ligaments, tendons, organs, skin, hair, and nails. Over time, your body doesn't replenish your collagen as quickly and that's a huge reason why you can look and feel older. READ MORE HERE; www.itsnotyourfaultyouvebeenliedto.com/book-bonuses/

TO SEE WHY, SCAN THE QR CODE BELOW
OR GO TO

WWW.ITSNOTYOURFAULTYOUVEBEENLIEDTO.COM/
BOOK-BONUSES

Tying it All Together

After working with Stephanie, she started to see the light. By adding good fats, she knew she and her family were forming a stronger foundation to keep their brains healthy. She understood which oils to cook with and which to avoid. She saw how the sugar she thought she was avoiding was showing up in her potatoes, rice, pasta, and bread. She made sure to add more vegetables. She even found that despite buying more expensive produce, her family's food bill went down because they didn't have to eat as much to feel full.

Two habits she found particularly effective were focusing on ADDITION instead of SUBTRACTION, as well as EATING ON SMALLER PLATES. By adding more nutrient dense foods to the foods she was currently eating, she found herself more satiated and less likely to reach for snacks or unhealthy foods throughout the day. As she got her energy back and built momentum, she was more able to resist and avoid the unhealthy foods she had been trying to remove from her diet for years. Eating from smaller plates served to reduce the total amount of calories she was able to consume while still tricking her brain into thinking she had eaten a full plate of food and would be satisfied. Those Okinawans sure know how to keep a brain and body sharp!

Further victories came in part by taking a higher quality supplement and making sure she and her family weren't eating to replace nutrients. Instead, they were eating only when they ACTUALLY needed energy. She noticed her hips slimming, and she could feel ribs where she hadn't felt ribs in a long time. Best of all, she felt more confident knowing that she was feeding herself and her family foods she KNEW were good for them. There was no more guesswork.

The truth is that nutrition doesn't need to be difficult. If you focus on the right principles, you're going to come out with the right answers.

Best of all, when you take the time to learn what your body really needs to be healthy, it's going to become a habit that you can pass on to your kids. The fact of the matter is the quality of the food the average person eats is continuing to diminish, and their ability to resist this trend in the culture around them will come from the habits and knowledge that's trained into them as they grow. This way, they know how to make the best decisions when it comes to choosing the healthiest foods to eat and how to avoid being tricked and deceived.

Marketers and big agribusiness are becoming more slick and clever all the time. They're finding new ways to use toxic chemicals and manipulate labels to keep you in the dark. Become ROCK SOLID on principles! By becoming rock solid on principles, you and your family will always be protected. You'll be far more likely to sort out how to eat the healthiest food.

Best of all, you'll know how to support your body with the best fuel so you can stay healthy and strong. You don't want to grow old and sick like the majority of people. Investing in healthy food is one of the best things you can do for you and your family.

TO COME TO A REAL FOOD FIESTA AND LEARN FOR YOURSELF HOW TO MAKE ANY UNHEALTHY RECIPE SUPER HEALTHY WITHOUT IT TASTING LIKE STICKS OR COSTING A FORTUNE, <u>SCAN THE QR CODE</u> BELOW FOR YOUR BONUSES OR GO TO

WWW.ITSNOTYOURFAULTYOUVEBEENLIEDTO.COM/ BOOK-BONUSES

Chapter 3
Exercise – Movement For Life

"Consistency is far better than rare moments of greatness."
– Scott Ginsberg

After seeing the title of this section, you're most likely having one of two reactions. Either you're excited to learn how to make your exercise and movement more effective, or you're absolutely dreading the idea of getting sweaty on a regular basis. Whichever reaction you felt, there's good news ahead.

For the exercise lovers, I'm going to show you a simple way to easily kick your exercises up a notch and make gains in power, flexibility, stamina, coordination, and balance all at the same time.

For those who despise exercise, I'll show you how to get it out of the way in only 9 – 15 minutes per day, at home, for little money, away from prying eyes, and still get all those benefits I just mentioned. Sounds like a good deal, doesn't it?

Here's why we have to talk about it. Movement is life. Anything that's not moving in some way is dead. There's no way around it, no matter how much you try to convince yourself otherwise. That's why we're going to talk about the most effective way to exercise so you can do what you need to do quickly, then get on with your day.

First, why is movement so necessary? To explain that, I'm going to bring out my inner geek for a second.

Your body is literally powered by gravity. You harness the power of gravity; the only constant force that you ever experience in this world. It powers your brain. Think of your brain as a computer, which can only work and send out commands to your body if it's powered up. No juice going up to your brain means no power to think and create, or send instructions to keep your organs and muscles working properly.

Your brain gets powered by nerve impulses coming up from your body largely as a result of your constant fight against gravity to stay upright. In every single muscle, you have mechanoreceptors and proprioceptors that register tiny changes in muscle length as you waver and correct in Earth's gravitational field.[19] These tiny changes in muscle length turn into a series of messages sending information to your brain, which keeps it healthy and energized. This forms a baseline of activation that provides the power to drive every higher, more evolved mental ability or process you're capable of. The amazing part is that EVERY SINGLE HIGHER MENTAL PROCESS IS BUILT ON THIS FOUNDATION OF NERVE IMPULSES THAT COME FROM FIGHTING GRAVITY. How cool is that???

That means your ability to think through problems, talk with your friends, dream about your future, remember events from your past, or experience the beauty of the moment is dependent on motion in your body. If there was no gravity, your brain would degrade in a hurry. That's why astronauts in space need to do resistance exercises regularly. The neurons in their brain die off rapidly when they're not actively resisting and moving in a gravity environment.[20]

With the rise of technology, you've been sold the lie that moving your body, staying active, and sweating are no longer necessary because machines do most of the work. When you look at the world's healthiest people, you see how they design their life around regular physical activity. They're always moving.

The shepherds of Sardinia are tough people who spend the majority of their day walking up and down hills with their livestock. The Seventh Day Adventists set aside an ENTIRE day devoted to family and nature walks.[7] They've learned over time that movement is life.

Activity is not an option; it's a requirement. While it's true that manual labor and physical jobs are less prevalent, the need to stay active regularly hasn't changed. The workplace may have changed, but the needs of your body haven't.

Now I understand that your job may have you at a desk or standing for 8+ hours a day, and you may feel it's impossible for you to structure your day to get that much activity, but don't give up hope. I'll show you how to keep your body healthy and active without quitting your job and becoming a shepherd.

And yes, it fits perfectly into your lifestyle, whether you travel, own a business, are a complete beginner, or have a family.

Stephanie had fallen into the trap of a modern, sedentary lifestyle and saw no way out of it. She'd become accustomed to using technology in her job and at home to make chores less physical. She remembered her mom having to use her body a lot more to get things done at home, but modern conveniences made everything easier for Stephanie.

She tried to make time to exercise on a regular basis, but was always so tired that her workouts often got pushed to the side. She was frustrated because she was too tired and busy to workout, even though she remembered how good she felt when she stayed active consistently.

Going to the gym took too much time out of her day, and she hadn't been able to find an at-home program that fit her busy schedule. She was frustrated because her weight had been creeping up for a long time, which made the pain and lack of energy even worse for her.

The idea that exercise and movement are less important in our technologically advanced society has even crept into schools. In an effort to free up classroom time for more advanced classes, gym class and sports are often seen as less important. Nothing could be further from the truth.

Kids need exercise and regular activity to drive and control the explosive growth of their brain and body during these crucial years.[21] This can literally be the difference between building a foundation of health or a foundation of illness as they get older.

Did you know that kids under the age of 5 are now the fastest growing segment of the non-adult population being prescribed antidepressants?[22] Between 1995 and 1999, antidepressant use increased 580% in the under 6 population and 151% in the 7–12 age group. In 2004, the FDA ordered that a "black box" label be placed on antidepressants warning that they can cause suicide in children and adolescents.[22]

Did you know that aerobic exercise has been found to be just as effective as Zoloft in treating major depression? According to a 1999 study reported in the Archives of Internal Medicine, 60-70% of participants were no longer classified as having major depression at the end of the 16 week study.[23] This was from simple exercise, without antidepressant medication and the laundry list of side-effects that accompany them.

Simple exercise keeps your brain stimulated and makes it more able to break negative feedback loops inside the brain. It naturally elevates your mood.

The bottom line is, if you want to be smarter, have better recall, and process emotions better, you had better keep your body moving, because your brain is dependent on motion to keep it powered up. If you're not moving, think of the battery in your brain slowly dying.

Imagine your cell phone with only 10% battery life left. You know you can't do a lot before it dies. Well, if you're not moving, it's like your brain is running with a low battery, struggling and trying to do its best. It's running out of juice. If you want to keep healthy, you have to move your body on a regular basis.

If I said the word "exercise" to you, what images would come to mind? Maybe you'd picture someone out for a morning run or jogging on a treadmill. Maybe you'd picture a muscled man or woman picking up heavy things and putting them down. Maybe you'd imagine an hour-long yoga class. Maybe you'd imagine a competitive game of football or basketball.

If you ask people to describe what exercise means to them, you'll usually get some variation of the above. That can definitely work, and if you love those activities, that's perfect. Keep doing them.

However, you may feel like you can't devote the kind of time for an hour-long run. Maybe you're out of shape and a competitive game would be downright exhausting and put you out of commission for a few days. Maybe you're intimidated by all the complex equipment at the gym and embarrassed that everyone but you seems to know what they're doing.

If so, I have a simple solution for you that will allow you to stay healthy at home in a short amount of time. Not only that, but it will grow with you as you get stronger and more fit. You'll learn about it a little later in this chapter.

For those of you who exercise regularly and think that what I'm about to show you will be a cake-walk, think again. This type of exercise is regularly used to train Olympic athletes, and I've personally seen them grimacing and struggling in the middle of this type of workout. It's tough.

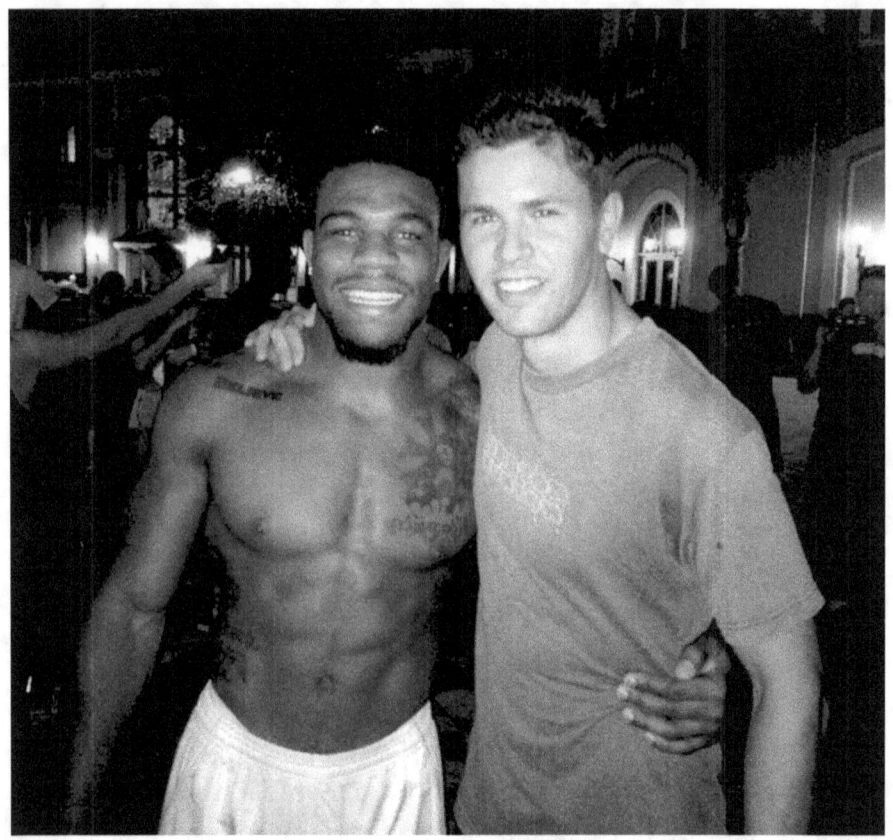

Olympic gold medallist Jordan Burroughs and I
after a 12 minute butt-kicking workout.

Better Than Cardio and Weights?

When you think of traditional cardio, what does that usually look like? In most cases, it involves using the treadmill, elliptical, or Stairmaster for 20 minutes to an hour. Over time, you hope that it'll be enough to help you lose weight, get your energy back, and give you the transformation you're working your butt off to get.

The problem with traditional cardio is that it's not the most effective. You only continue to burn fat for approximately 30 minutes after you're done working out.[24] That's okay, but I'll show you a way to get better results.

The other issue with cardio is that is raises cortisol and stress hormones, which break down muscle over time. This is bad for a couple reasons.

Stress hormones keep your body in a constant state of "fight or flight" meaning you never get a chance to fully heal and repair from the stress of your day.[25] Over time, the damage from the day builds up, which can cause problems with sore joints, inflammation, slow healing, etc.

The other reason is that as you age, your body naturally loses muscle tissue, so the LAST thing you want to do is exercise in a way that's going to accelerate that process.[25] Cardio has also been shown to be a very poor way of losing weight.[26]

Don't worry. I'm not going to leave you hanging. The good news is on its way!

At this point, you're probably wondering why the exercise I'll show you is so good. Here's why. First off, it's more natural. This type of exercise is primarily done with body weight, and builds real ability in your body much faster. That means your body is stronger. It has better balance. It's more coordinated. It allows you to keep your independence longer.

One of the most dangerous events that can happen as you get older is a simple fall. Quite often it's life-threatening, or threatens your independence or ability to live alone inside your own home. That means anything you can do to improve strength and balance will help keep you out of the old folks' home or the morgue.

This type of exercise also stabilizes your spine and joints better than traditional cardio because it's more dynamic. It builds your stamina and cardiovascular endurance faster. It's a whole body exercise that's more in-line with how we've used our bodies for thousands of years. It also allows your body to burn fat for 24-36 hours AFTER you're done exercising. How sweet is that??

If you're looking to bulk up, you can easily add a weight vest, ankle weights, or dumbbells to make it more challenging and allow you to build muscle.

If that wasn't enough, this exercise shapes and changes how your hormones are expressed in your body.[27] This is a HUGE advantage if you want to stay healthy as you get older. Your hormones are either your best friend or your worst enemy. If they're on your side, getting fit almost becomes automatic. If they're not, you're in for a real battle.

Here's how it works. Your body has two primary sources of fuel: sugar and fat. Your hormones prime your body to primarily burn one or the other in response to whichever fuel you give it to work with. Most people are loaded with sugar, so their hormones are set up to make the process of burning sugar faster and more efficient. However, this is not good if you want to stay healthy your whole life.

With the exercise I'm going to show you, you exhaust your sugar supply and force your body to fire up the fat-burning pathways, allowing you to melt through excess fat like it's going out of style. This is why you'll be burning fat for up to 36 hours AFTER YOU FINISH WORKING OUT.[27]

This exercise has shown itself to be fantastic for diabetics and pre-diabetics because it fires up the machinery inside your cells and helps to reduce insulin resistance.[27] Diabetes highly predisposes you to develop secondary cancers. The high amount of blood sugar caused by diabetes is the primary fuel that cancer MUST HAVE to survive and gain a foothold in your body. If you've been dealing with diabetes, this has been shown to be one of the best exercises you can do.

This exercise also stimulates human growth hormone (HGH) and testosterone.[27]

The benefits just keep coming with this exercise, because it'll fit perfectly into your busy schedule. Instead of the normal hour to 90 minute workouts, you can be done in as little as 9 minutes. How great is that? 9 minutes!

Where most people are getting older and slower, with less energy and more disease, you'll be getting your life and energy back in spades! You'll be able to do the things that you love without tearing your body apart or having to pay for it for days afterwards.

Show Me This Magical Exercise

Enough teasing! What's this exercise called?

You may know it as high intensity interval training (HIIT), burst training, or surge training. In essence, it gives you the privilege of working out at YOUR maximum for a short interval—20 seconds, 30 seconds, or a minute—followed by a short rest. The key that makes it so POWERFUL is you must give it everything you've got for the short interval you're working out.

With that said, it's important to know that everyone starts at different levels, so you're only competing with yourself. Listen to your body. If it hurts, slow down or modify the exercise. Find a qualified chiropractor, physiotherapist, and massage therapist to help condition and rehab your body as you push through new exercises.

HIIT is a multi-joint, multi-muscle exercise that mimics natural movements. You're going to be building muscle in coordination, where activation of one muscle feeds into activation of another, into another, into another. This creates a beautiful dance where you build functional strength so you can use your body.

What I LOVE about this exercise is that I can do it rain or shine in a living room, playground, office, hotel room, cabin, campground, or wherever I happen to find myself. It takes any excuse I might have for not exercising and throws it right out the window. For you, it'll do the same.

Let's See It in Action

A couple weeks after getting started with Stephanie, she finally had her pain levels down to the point where she wanted to know what exercises she could do to help her lose weight and get her energy back. She was thrilled with the idea that she could workout for only 9 minutes a day and still see results. Although she was a little skeptical at the beginning, she decided she had nothing to lose and tried it.

When she came back to my office two days later, she was amazed at how intense the exercise was. Even though it was only 9 minutes, she found she couldn't finish it. Her whole body was sore but she loved how it made her feel. Over the next few weeks, she did the exercise 3-4 times per week consistently and was amazed at how quickly she found her energy returning.

Her body started to feel energized and she was sleeping better. Overall, her mood started to lift and the tasks that seemed to take so much out of her just a few weeks before seemed to hardly bother her now. She was down about 8 pounds and excited to keep going. She said to me, "If this is how good I feel after a few weeks, I can't wait to see how good I'll feel a few months from now!"

At this point you may be saying, "Yeah, yeah, yeah, let's see it in action." Don't worry, I have you covered. Below is a routine I prepared for you that you can do anywhere. We made sure to avoid shooting the video in a gym without any equipment just to show you how simple it is. When you watch it, remember that I've been doing it for quite some time, so start where you are and be gracious with yourself. You'll get stronger with time.

TO SEE HIGH INTENSITY INTERVAL TRAINING IN ACTION
SCAN THE QR CODE BELOW
OR GO TO

WWW.ITSNOTYOURFAULTYOUVEBEENLIEDTO.COM/
BOOK-BONUSES

Chapter 4
Toxicity – Poisons.
Poisons Everywhere

"What you put in your body can either be the most powerful form of medicine or the slowest form of poison."

– Ann Wigmore

Let's talk about toxins.

It will come as a surprise to exactly no one that to live a healthy life, you need to reduce your exposure to toxins and chemicals. This isn't exactly rocket-science.

The difficulty in avoiding them comes from the fact that they're everywhere. They're in and on your food. They're in your personal care products. They're in your household cleaners. They're in the water. They're in the air. They're in your clothes. They're in fragrances. They're in the products that you use to take care of your kids. There's never been a time in human history where you've been surrounded by so many chemicals and foreign agents.

They're sold by slick marketers who tell you they've solved your problems through chemistry. If you have a stain, there's a product that can remove it. If you have a problem, there's a new plastic machine that'll fix it. If you have an illness, there's a pill that will suppress it. If you have a pan that sticks, have I got an answer for you!

There's an endless array of new fragrances, cleaners, medications, additives, herbicides, etc. designed to make our lives EASIER. Almost all of them involve toxic chemicals that don't occur naturally anywhere in nature.

You're told these chemicals have been tested and they won't hurt you, or the effect is so minimal it'll never affect you in any meaningful way. And so you trust them.

However, just because a solution to a problem of yours is easier, does not always make it better.

The reality is your body has never been under such a toxic load in the history of humankind. It's become obvious these chemicals ARE affecting us in serious ways.

For example, it seems more and more people are finding it more difficult to lose weight now despite changing their diet and exercising regularly. This is hugely frustrating. Think of how much effort it takes to research recipes, make healthy meals, pack them ahead of and then, at the end of the day, you see no changes.

Here's where many people accept the lie that getting healthy isn't possible for them. They believe they're too old. They've been cursed with bad genes. They don't have the willpower.

It's not true.

You've been fed a lie and have been beating yourself up ever since. Remember, you need the right information and the right support to make a lasting change. Celebrate your effort and don't beat yourself up.

When your body encounters toxins or synthetic chemicals it can't process, it often makes the choice to sequester and store those toxins in your fat cells rather than allow them to continue to circulate in your body. This is an intelligent choice because your body knows those toxins can't be allowed to float around in your bloodstream. As a result, it stores them in your fat.

When you start exercising, hoping to lose the extra weight, your body says, "I can't let you burn this fat because you'll release the toxins. Sorry, not going to happen." You have to take the steps to clear out the toxins before your body will let you burn the fat.

Another huge problem we face is from plastics. The chemicals used to make plastics flexible (like BPA) mimic our natural hormones. They're called "xenoestrogens." When they get absorbed into your body through your hands, or through food that comes in contact with them, they raise the levels of estrogen in your body.

Elevated estrogen is linked to all kinds of cancers, especially female or hormone-driven cancers like cervical cancer, breast cancer, and uterine cancer.[28] One of estrogen's jobs is to make cells divide faster, which is why it's found in higher concentrations in women. This makes sense considering rapid cell division is how uterine linings grow and babies develop. When you raise the levels of estrogen in your body, cells divide faster, increasing your chance of developing and accelerating tumor growth.

The problem compounds because your body has a hard time getting rid of these chemicals once they're inside you. They build up and accumulate in your cells and poison your body. While it's impossible for you to avoid these chemicals completely, you can make simple changes to eliminate the largest sources of toxins that are affecting the health of you and your family.

This was another side of Stephanie's frustration. She had been fit growing up, but found that it was becoming increasingly hard to lose weight when she exercised. Prior to meeting me, her workout routine was sporadic. She noticed it had become more of a chore to lose the weight she put on around the holidays or family gatherings. Imagine her frustration when she would try her best to eat well and exercise, and still wouldn't see her body change.

When we talked about how all the chemicals in her home are absorbed and stored in her body, a light bulb went off in her head. This was something she'd never considered, in her mind, the chemicals she bought at the store couldn't be that dangerous. After all, why would they be available for sale if they were so dangerous?

She was eager to get rid of the chemicals in her house, not just for her health, but for the health of her husband and daughters. At the same time, she was apprehensive that the natural cleaners I showed her would not be effective at getting things clean like she was used to. She also was concerned that making her own cleaners would be difficult or time-consuming and would put a strain on her already full schedule.

Reluctantly, she decided to start slowly, eliminating the traditional cleaners she bought at the store as each one ran out, and replacing them with natural cleaners made with ingredients she could actually pronounce and spell.

I'm Toxic! Now What?

Think of your body as simply a collection of cells inside one big community. Each of your 70 trillion cells interacts with the other cells around it to stay informed, protected, and working together. When your cells are healthy, your body is healthy.

Now think of these cells as buckets instead. 70 trillion buckets! You either put good things into your 70 trillion buckets or you put toxic things in them. The way most of us are living, we're slowly filling up these buckets with toxic chemicals. When these buckets are full of chemicals, it's impossible for you to be healthy.

You may be asking yourself, "What can I do if these chemicals are everywhere?"

The answer has two parts:

1. **Stop filling your buckets**
2. **Empty your full buckets**

I know, it's rocket science.

1. Stop filling your buckets

Yes, toxins are everywhere, and we can never avoid them all, but don't give up. Even if you were to make one change and stick with it, that's a great place to grow from. To make it easier, I'm going to show you the largest sources of toxins, and simple solutions that you can do to stop filling your body with these very common, easy-to-eliminate toxins.

A. **Household cleaning products** – Buy natural, chemical-free cleaners, or make your own in bulk.
B. **Pesticides and herbicides** – Prioritize which foods to buy organic with the Environmental Working Group's Clean 15 and Dirty Dozen list.
C. **Steroids, growth hormones, and antibiotics** – Buy free range organic chicken and grass fed beef. Consider buying a quarter or half a cow with another family.
D. **Preservatives, additives, and colorings** – Only buy foods with ingredients you can pronounce or spell, and that sound like something that would grow in nature.
E. **Teflon cookware** – Buy stainless steel or ceramic. The non-stick features are not worth the damage from the harsh chemicals that give pans their non-stick abilities.

F. **Tap water** – Filter your water or get a water purifier that doesn't strip out the minerals.

G. **Personal care products** – Switch to natural products without the chemicals.

H. **Heavy metals** from things like Atlantic fish, mercury (silver) fillings, paint, etc. – Avoid these things where possible.

I. **Bio-toxins (mold)** – Seek out certified professionals and specialized natural physicians.

J. **Medications** – Use the rest of the strategies in this book to get healthy naturally. Most of the diseases we face now are caused by our lifestyle. As you change the way you live, the need for this medication to mask the symptoms can disappear. Work with your doctors to take as few medications as possible.

Source: Lerner, Ben, et al. Maximized Living Makeover. Maximized Living Publishing. Orlando, Florida. 2008.

Again, be gracious with yourself. Start small and grow from there.

Each change I felt in my body motivated me to do greater. It also made me re-evaluate the way I'd been living my life, and made me question whether every modern convenience actually contributed to my life or stole from it. I came to the conclusion that making myself sick or stealing my energy was not a worthwhile trade-off to make certain jobs easier or faster.

As a bonus, I don't have to live like the Amish either. I just have to think differently. There's something to be said for following the timeless ways of doing things, even if they're not always the most efficient. When it comes to putting toxins in your body, there's always a price to pay.

Let's see how Stephanie did with the process.

When we first talked about removing sources of toxicity, she was understandably skeptical whether she could switch from products she'd known all her life. She raised all kinds of objections about cost, time, and difficulty. When she found out how she could clean her whole house with just water and some simple and inexpensive ingredients, and then slowly change the products she used as each ran out, she became more receptive.

Over the next few months, her confidence grew, and she loved the idea of having a house that was completely safe for her family without the chemical residue. Mixing her own cleaners had become second nature for her, and she was slightly embarrassed at having put up such a fight in the beginning.

However, she was concerned about what to do about the toxins that were already inside her. How could she get those out?

2. Empty Your Buckets
It's a great thing to stop filling your buckets, but what about the toxins which are already there? It's no good to leave them in your cells, messing everything up.

Fortunately, your body has special detox pathways that can clear out the crud you've put into your body over the years. The main player in that system is a molecule called glutathione. Glutathione is a superhero in your body. It's like the quarterback. It tells every other player in your detoxification team exactly what to do.

Now think about your life and how much stress you're under. Think about all the times you've skipped meals or had fast food. Think of all the times you didn't get as much sleep as you wanted. Think of all the processed food you've ever eaten. Think of all the electromagnetic radiation you get from your phone and computer.

I'm sure you could create quite an extensive list.

The bottom line is that all of these stressors will harm your body in some way. It's glutathione's job to clear the toxins and damage, and build you back up again. With how fast your life moves, that's an exhausting job! Over time, your glutathione levels can become depleted.[29] When they get depleted, you have to build them back up again or else your whole detox team falls apart. With stress coming from all sides, that's a bad place to be.

On top of that, glutathione is a main driver of your immune system.[30] When you're feeling run down by the stress of life, so are your glutathione levels. Isn't it interesting that you often get sick when your body is feeling run down? Your glutathione levels and your immune system aren't up to the task of fighting off the germs and bacteria, and those invaders are able to get a foothold in your body. This creates disease.

Glutathione is unique. You can't eat glutathione or take a glutathione supplement to replenish your levels. Your stomach destroys glutathione when you eat it. However, you CAN eat foods that contain the building blocks of glutathione. This is where the latest push with antioxidants comes from. The more you get into your body, the better you'll be able to repair and recover from the stresses of your day.

The onslaught you face on a daily basis is increasing in intensity. The amount of chemicals, radiation, poor nutrition, lack of sleep, distractions, medications, etc. has never been higher, meaning your glutathione levels are more taxed than ever before.

It's become more difficult to keep your glutathione levels where they need to be given the nutrient content in today's food and the amount of stress you face every day. It's a very difficult task. Your food doesn't have the nutrients it once had, and the stresses you face keep increasing.

For that reason, there are only a few specific glutathione boosters that are up to the task of enhancing your body's immune system and detoxification. These have been shown to boost your glutathione levels long term because of their ability to get the amino acid cysteine INTO your cells. This is vital because cysteine is the rate-limiting step in your body's ability to produce glutathione rapidly enough to protect you. There have even been pilot studies to determine whether products like these should be used in conjunction with chemotherapy in caring for people battling cancer.[31] This is because of their dramatic ability to restore or rebuild your immune system after chemotherapy decimates it. They're rockstars and worth checking out!

Your Body Is Not a Landfill

Stephanie had made great strides in creating a chemical-free house, and staying focused on which products will allow her to keep herself and her family safe. As of this writing, she has yet to fully start boosting her glutathione levels, but in consulting her physician, she sees it as a vital part of her overall plan. For now, she's concentrating on being diligent with the other choices she's made. However, she knows that in time, this will be part of her lifestyle too.

Keeping your cells healthy is essential if you want to be able to age without falling apart. Your body is not a landfill. You're worth more than a dumping ground for toxic chemicals. The more you keep your body clear of toxins, the better off you'll be.

Start by addressing the major sources of toxicity. It's easier than you think, and the amount of mental clarity and energy you can regain will be worth the work.

The next step is to clear out the junk you've been carrying with you for decades. You're worth it! Give your body the tools it needs to keep running clean and you'll have the best chance to live the kind of life you've long since thought was behind you.

TO GET YOUR COPY OF THE ENVIRONMENTAL WORKING
GROUP'S CLEAN 15/DIRTY DOZEN, TO LEARN MORE
ABOUT YOU CAN GET A BOOST FROM GLUTATHIONE,
AND TO CREATE YOUR OWN CHEMICAL FREE HOME
IN 2 WEEKS FOR LESS THAN $150,
SCAN THE QR CODE BELOW
OR GO TO

WWW.ITSNOTYOURFAULTYOUVEBEENLIEDTO.COM/
BOOK-BONUSES

Chapter 5
Nerve Supply – Your Spark
From Within

"The nervous system holds the key to the body's incredible potential to heal itself."

– Sir Jay Holder M.D., D.C., Ph.D.

Up to this point, we've talked about:

1. Mindset – Creating a true picture of yourself and your potential
2. Nutrition – The fuel that will keep your body running tip-top your whole life
3. Exercise – Why motion is life, and how simple it is to get it daily
4. Toxicity – Cutting out poisons that steal from your life

These pillars are all fantastic, but they're all secondary. Let me show you what I mean.

Imagine this scenario with me.

If a person who had passed away just 5 minutes ago was laying in front of you, and you put the best food into him, would it do him any good? No, of course not.

If you hooked his body up to a machine and moved it or did exercise for him, would it help? No.

If you made sure his body wasn't exposed to chemicals, would it make any difference at all? Silly question. Of course not.

The point here is that ULTIMATELY, health is NOT an OUTSIDE-IN thing. True health always comes from the INSIDE-OUT. It's not the food or exercise that makes you healthy. It's your body's ability to use it which does. This ability requires a spark and a force inside you, which allows your body to live and rebuild. There is no other way.

When Stephanie and I first talked, this was what she found most intriguing. The idea that her body is designed to heal made so much sense to her, but she never gave any real thought to how she could support it in that way. She thought diet and exercise were all she needed to be healthy.

After our first session, she came away with a full understanding of what it takes to make sure her body could work and heal the way it was supposed to. For the first time in a long time, she had hope that the nagging injuries and pains that wouldn't go away despite other forms of treatment, could actually clear up and heal.

Unfortunately, our healthcare system is not built to focus on the INSIDE-OUT method of healing. What we have in North America is an OUTSIDE-IN approach to health.

You're told that as you get older, your body is less able to fend off the aches, pains, diseases, and effects of aging. It's inevitable for your body to break down after years of hard use, abuse, poor diet, little exercise, and the accumulation of chemicals. There's little difference you can make by trying to live an active, healthy lifestyle because studies show that none of these isolated things you do can definitely stop your body from developing disease or becoming unhealthy.

But don't worry! There are medicines that can block and disguise any symptom of any disease so that you don't have to change your lifestyle. You can continue to live the exact same way that allowed the problem to develop in the first place. And if that doesn't work, modern medicine can always get you back to health by cutting out whichever part of your body isn't working right.

Our medical system views the solution to disease from the viewpoint of giving you medicine to remove the symptoms of the disease you're facing, or doing surgery if the problem becomes bad enough. They spend less time educating you on how to address the root causes of why you're sick or in pain.

Unleash the Power Inside You

I'm going to show you how your body is incredibly intelligent, and will always work to create health from the INSIDE-OUT if given the opportunity to.

What do I mean by that?

What I mean is the lifeless body in our earlier example had all the same parts as you or I, but it's missing that one thing that gives us life. It's missing that spark.

That spark is what tells your heart to beat and your lungs to take in oxygen. It's what tells your stomach and digestive organs how to digest your food. It's what tells your body parts how to heal if they get injured. It drives all your detox pathways to make sure you're cleaning the crud out of your body. It's why you have dreams, emotions, language, relationships, and movement. It's the reason you're alive. Without it, you're no different than the lifeless corpse in our example.

That spark is your nerve supply. It's your nervous system.

This is the power that animates your body. It's the signals from your brain down to your body, and from your body up to your brain. It's the intelligence that knows how to keep your body in perfect balance so you can stay healthy for life. It's the force that takes all the food, exercise, supplements, protein powders, sleep, water, and anything else you could possibly give your body and directs EXACTLY how your body uses them.

Without it, everything you learned about in the previous chapters is meaningless.

I'll show you how important your nervous system is.

- We all know food is important, yes? We can go weeks without taking in any food.
- We all know water is important, yes? We can go days without drinking a drop of water and still live.
- Oxygen is important, yes? We can go minutes without oxygen.
- However, your body cannot go one second without a proper nerve supply. Your brain must constantly send the right messages down to the rest of your body for you to stay alive and healthy.

Your nervous system is the first system in your body to form, and it's the one that directs and controls EVERY other process in your body. Nothing happens without it.[32]

Your Command Center

So what is your nervous system?

It's your brain, your spinal cord (which is inside the bones of your back), and your nerves. Your nerves are what send instructions from your brain down to your body, and send information from your body up to your brain. It's a continuous cycle that keeps your brain fully informed about the stresses your body is facing, allowing it to respond in the exact right way so you can stay healthy.

When your nerves are working properly, every part of your body does the exact right thing, at the right time, depending on the situation you find yourself in. If your nerves are unhealthy, your body doesn't always do the right thing, making it impossible to be healthy long term.

Protecting Your Command Center

Your body is smart. Since your nervous system is so vital, it makes sense to protect it. That's exactly what your body does. It surrounded your brain and spinal cord in bone to protect it, forming your skull and spinal column. Think body armor. Your skull and vertebrae protect your command center. However, it can't make these structures completely rigid or you wouldn't be able to move. Your spinal column is designed for protection AND movement.

This means your body works like a machine, where all the parts have to be in the right place for it to work properly. If the parts are exactly where they need to be, the machine works well and the parts last for a long time. If they're not, it's no good.

So how do you keep your nervous system healthy when no one showed you how or even told you how important it is?

There are 2 primary ways:

1. Motion
Your spine has to move to stay healthy. This is because the discs in between your vertebrae and the ligaments that hold it all together have very little blood supply.[33] Instead they get all their nutrition through motion. The constant motion of your spine moves nutrients in, and helps get waste products out.

To get a visual, think of the difference between a clear, running mountain stream where water is constantly replenished, as opposed to a dank, stinky, festering pond where no water moves in or out.

No good.

This is why the healthiest cultures in the world build their daily routines around regular movement and exercise. From the shepherds of Sardinia to the Seventh Day Adventists of Loma Linda, California, the people who live into their 90s and 100s most often build movement into their daily lives.[7]

The lack of motion in any joint is a major cause of arthritis. Maybe you've been told that arthritis is normal as you get older, or it runs in your family. These are more lies. While arthritis is common, it's absolutely not normal.

It's been shown that any joint in your body that isn't moving properly for more than 2 weeks suffers irreversible micro-damage.[33] The lack of proper motion prevents nutrition from getting to your discs and ligaments. The lack of proper motion is why they start to degenerate. Over time, the degeneration builds up, causing your joints to become less stable.

Your body looks at that unstable situation and says, "I can't have that kind of instability so close to my spinal cord." In response, it does the best thing it knows how. It starts to lay down bone to stabilize it. Those bony growths eventually cause the pain you know as arthritis.

This may be news for you. Unfortunately, what advice do you often hear from health professionals?

"Here's some Tylenol or Advil and muscle relaxants. Take them and you'll be fine."

What good is pain medication or a muscle relaxant for you to actually fix the problem when the issue is not tight muscles, but a lack of proper motion in the joints of your spine?

Instead of covering up the symptoms, I'm going to show you a simple way to get proper motion into your spine, whether you sit at a desk, stand at an assembly line, or are very physical with your body all day.

It's a 5 minute exercise you can do anywhere to help you get all the nutrients you need into your discs to keep them healthy and reduce your chance of developing arthritis as you get older. This exercise will also fire up your nerves to keep you awake when you get tired or fatigued from sitting too long.

This was one of the most important exercises to stabilize Stephanie's spine and make sure that she was able to get better as quickly as possible. Taking care of her family as well as her mom put a major strain on her family's budget, so the exercises she was able to do helped her to see maximum benefit from each of our sessions.

She saw faster progress and longer lasting results. She found that her brain quickly fired up once she started to do these exercises too. Not only that, but her core was tighter as well.

TO SEE EXACTLY WHAT THE SPINAL STABILIZATION
EXERCISES LOOK LIKE, SCAN THE QR CODE BELOW
OR GO TO

WWW.ITSNOTYOURFAULTYOUVEBEENLIEDTO.COM/
BOOK-BONUSES

2. Alignment

Your spine has a normal alignment to it which allows it to fully protect and support your nerves, WHILE allowing your body to move and bend as you need it to. Your spine should be completely straight when viewed from the front, with three separate curves when viewed from the side.

These curves are incredibly important. Without them, there's tension and pressure in your spinal cord and nerves where they leave your spinal canal between the bones of your back.

In your neck, you're supposed to have a curve between 35 and 45 degrees with the convex side of the curve pointing forward.[34] Think of it like a letter C. When your spine is in the proper alignment, your spinal cord can drape nicely inside the spinal canal without any pressure on it.

However, it's very common for your head to shift forward, which eliminates the natural curve in your neck. This causes the bones in your neck to be straight instead of following that proper C-shaped curve. This can be a result of traumas like car accidents, or daily, repetitive activities like texting, slouching, watching TV, sleeping with tall pillows, or anything else that pushes your head forward. Look around at all the people constantly looking down at their phones or computers. When your neck straightens out, it puts tension and pressure on your spinal cord and affects the delicate nerves that control every organ in your body.

Stephanie was shocked at what her X-rays showed. Not only did she not have a C-curve in her neck, it was slightly reversed and leaning forward. She couldn't believe there could be that much damage to her spine when she didn't have a significant amount of pain in her neck. I explained that pain is almost always the last symptom to show up whenever there's a problem. Your body has an amazing ability to deal with problems below the surface without you even being aware of it, but eventually, any problem becomes too much, and that's when you notice symptoms and pain.

Years of damage from poor posture and a few minor car accidents could easily explain how her neck could be in such bad shape. She asked if the poor alignment could have been due to the position she was in when the X-ray was taken. I told her it was unlikely because of the significant amount of degeneration and arthritis in her neck. She was shocked.

"How could there be arthritis in my neck?? I'm not THAT old!"

I explained that just like a car wheel that's out of alignment wears out faster, bones in her spine start to degenerate and develop arthritis when they're out of position. The bones above and below were fine despite being the exact same age. However, the bones most affected by poor posture and trauma had begun to "wear out", causing her pain and affecting the nerves that come out between the bones.

It's easy to be frustrated when you've been dealing with aches and pains that have slowly become worse over time, despite your best efforts to fix the problem. Maybe you're wondering why you have unusual symptoms in your body even though the tests of your organs comes back normal.

The issue may not be with the organs themselves, but rather the CONTROL of your organs that keep them from working and repairing the way they should. By looking at the health of your nerve system and making sure the position of your spine isn't contributing to your problems, you may be able to improve the root cause of your issues.

Unfortunately, you may not have ever heard any of this nervous system talk. You likely only hear your nervous system mentioned in the context of full-blown neurological conditions like Multiple Sclerosis. However, the research is there.

Forward head posture puts up to 40 pounds of pressure on your delicate spinal cord.[35] That's how much pressure is in your car's tires, which support your 4000 pound car! This can cause major problems with the autonomic (think automatic) nervous system. This is the part of your nervous system that regulates all your body processes that run in the background without you having to think about them. When you think of your autonomic nervous system, think of your heart beat, digestion, balance, immune system, hormones, etc. You know, the important stuff.

It works like this for every organ, cell, and tissue that your nerves supply. Any nerve or bundle of nerves that is affected by the poor alignment of your spine will not be able to send the proper messages to the various parts of your body working properly.

For instance, your neck, shoulder, upper back muscles, thyroid gland, heart, lungs, head, face, and jaw are all supplied by the nerves in your neck or upper back. Pressure on these nerves can contribute to headaches, migraines, neck pain, shoulder problems, numbness and tingling in your arms, muscle weakness or fatigue, balance problems, ringing in the ears, or poor sleep.

Quite the list!

One of the best things you can do for your health long term is to protect your posture. The simplest way to do that is to stand or sit with good posture. To practice proper posture, here's a simple way to remember it:

- Suck your belly button towards your spine (Think sucking in your stomach)
- Bring your shoulders back and down (Think of tucking your shoulder blades into your back pockets)

- Press your head up against an imaginary ceiling to lengthen your spine and engage your stabilizing muscles
- Lightly press your ankles towards each other to engage your big glute (butt) muscles (flex)

Another thing you can do is to make sure you protect the natural C-shaped curve in your neck. Here's how:

- Not slouching when watching TV
- Bringing your phone up to eye level when texting
- Propping up your laptop, computer monitor, or textbooks
- Sleeping with few/thin pillows
- Working at a stand-up workstation
- Avoiding looking down for long periods of time

I Think My Body is Broken. What Do I Do?

You may be saying, "That's great, but I don't do any of those things you just mentioned and I know my posture sucks. What can I do?"

The best thing you can do is have your spine and nerves checked by a chiropractor. Even if the bones of your back have been out of alignment or not moving properly for a long time, you'd be surprised at the kind of transformation that can happen. An adjustment is your first step towards better health because of its effect on the health of your nerves, as well as the joints of your body. You may be tempted to start with another modality or therapy, but I'll show you why your first step should be adjustments to restore the proper function to your nerves and relieve any irritation caused by inflammation of your joints.

That's not to say other therapies aren't necessary. They absolutely are, and very important for you to heal at your best, but relieving the pressure in your nervous system through adjustments is often the very first area of focus.

This is because your nervous system is primary. This is the first place to start because it will allow your body to heal. The injured area begins receiving the proper instructions regarding how to direct the healing process. This way, any other therapy you seek out will be more effective and long-lasting.

The adjustment is a technique that's been used for thousands of years across many different cultures.[37] Traditional "bonesetters" were sought out to heal people from all sorts of disorders. Even Hippocrates, the father of modern medicine, said "look well to the spine for the cause of all disease." He understood that the nervous system is primary, and that any issue with your nerves would ultimately show up in your organs.

This was shown in 1931 by Dr. Henry Winsor, who found that disease in an organ could nearly always be related to the nerves that supplied that organ.[38] This is profound because we've known the effect of the nervous system in creating or healing the body for so long, yet this may be the very first you've heard something like this. Dr. Winsor found that "there was nearly a 100% correlation between minor curvature of the spine and diseases of the internal organs."[38]

That's huge! Read that again.

I realize that some people have had bad experiences with a chiropractor before, and that's unfortunate. Bear with me and you'll find a way to make sure your spine and nerves stay healthy, while making sure you're comfortable with the whole process.

Chiropractic can be a very polarizing profession. However, looking at how your nervous system works and how important spinal alignment and motion is to your overall health, everyone DOES need to visit a chiropractor to keep your spine and nerves healthy. This allows you to keep your body working at its best over the long term.

The question then becomes "how do we improve your spinal alignment and nervous system health in a way that you're comfortable with?" You need to fully understand what's happening at all times so there's no confusion.

In my experience, the biggest reason why someone had a negative experience with a chiropractor is because there was a miscommunication about what was happening or what to expect. The chiropractor may have explained the situation and solution, but that doesn't mean it was said in a way that connected with you, the patient. You or the chiropractor could have been rushed or preoccupied that day. There may not have been a deep level of connection. Any number of things could have happened.

This makes it extremely important to find a chiropractor who will take the time to explain exactly what's happening in your spine and nerves, and to make sure you're comfortable and fully informed every step of the way.

The first step is to have an open, honest conversation so that you both can get onto the same page. You need to talk about the specifics of what's been happening, what results you want to see, what's worked well or poorly in the past, and what roadblocks you can see that may stop you from getting the results you want.

The next step is a detailed assessment that will look at:

- Range of motion
- Flexibility
- Posture
- The health of your nerves
- The health and condition of your joints and muscles
- The alignment and motion of your spine
- Orthopedic and neurological testing

Once we have a full understanding of what's going on with you, and what results you want, then we can go to work putting together a custom-tailored plan to improve the health of your spine and nervous system.

If you're concerned about the adjustment hurting, don't be. There are many ways to get the job done without any popping sounds. There are spring-loaded instruments, stretches, and exercises that are gentle but effective, in addition to the traditional methods of adjusting.

The benefit of a chiropractic adjustment is that chiropractors are specially trained to be very specific with their adjustment. This means that the adjustment focuses on improving motion and alignment of the affected joint, rather than a generalized manipulation of a general region. By doing that, your joints become less inflamed and begin to heal properly. The irritation to your nerve roots begin to decrease.

The most important aspect of the adjustment is taking the pressure off your nerves so you can fully express your health from within.

This is especially important for kids. Their brain and body develop so quickly, and they're always falling and hurting themselves. It's much easier to keep kids healthy than to fix sick and stiff adults.

The adjustments for kids are very gentle. They use about the same pressure as you'd use to check a tomato for ripeness. When the problems haven't been there as long, it's so much easier to correct them. The healthier their nervous system is, the better opportunity for them to grow into the fabulous young people that they're designed to be, without anything holding them back.

In addition to adjustments, any approach needs to be done in conjunction with specific exercises to stabilize and strengthen the small but incredibly important muscles and ligaments that support your spine.

This way you get better quicker, spend less money, see lasting changes, and give yourself the best chance of staying strong and healthy your whole life. It's no fun when you feel like you're going to a professional time and time again and not seeing results. No one has time for that.

Let's come back to Stephanie.

Over the last couple months, she's made amazing strides at improving both the alignment and movement of her spine. In addition to the adjustments, she's been doing her spinal stabilization exercises faithfully and has taken steps to make her work environment more conducive to protecting the curve in her neck.

The arthritis pain she had felt in her neck has started to improve, and the soreness in her wrists and shoulders has gone down as the pressure has come off her nerves. She's also noticed that when she gets sick, she has more energy to recover and get back to feeling great. Even after a hard day, she has more energy, so she can take care of her family and still be able to enjoy her favorite activities again. Her knees, which had been a major headache for her, are getting better. They feel better than they have in the last 10 years.

Here's Your Summary

Health is an INSIDE-OUT process.

If you want to stay healthy, you have to take care of your nerves. Your nerves control how everything in your body heals and works over time.

You've been sold the lie that medicine or surgery are the only way to get you back to health. The most important step you can take is to make sure your brain can fully direct every part of your body. If you want to be able to stay young and do everything that you love to do, you have to take care of your nerves.

Taking care of your nerves means taking care of your spine. This is why chiropractic care is essential. When you keep your spine in the right alignment and moving properly, you're going to be miles ahead of most people. You'll continue to be healthy when everybody else is slowing down and giving up what they love.

If you feel like you've been out of the game for a long time, here's a fresh start. Take it and run with it, because no matter your age, your body can improve if you give it the opportunity to.

TO SEE THE SPECIFIC EXERCISES MY PRIVATE CLIENTS
USE TO BUILD LONG TERM STABILITY IN THEIR SPINES,
AND TO SEE WHAT YOU CAN EXPECT FROM YOUR FIRST
SESSION WITH ME, SCAN THE QR CODE BELOW
OR GO TO

WWW.ITSNOTYOURFAULTYOUVEBEENLIEDTO.COM/
BOOK-BONUSES

Chapter 6
The Complete Package

"Be strong enough to stand alone, smart enough to know when you need help, and brave enough to ask for it."

— Ziad K. Abdelnour

At this point, you have all the information you need to create strong, robust health and break free of the lies, misconceptions, and deceit that keep most people from being healthy. On top of that, you have the tools to do it in a way that's sustainable. It's worked for people who have lived these principles over thousands of years.

Before you get too excited, let me caution you. You've felt hopeful before, and more often than not, you've been let down. Roadblocks have stopped you from reaching the goals you set and limited your belief. Let's look at the challenges you face and how you can overcome them. Unless you face these barriers, you won't know how to push through them when they inevitably face you again.

The good news is you can overcome them. Health is yours for the taking. You just need the right information and the right support.

When Stephanie came to me, she had been ready for a change for years. She saw the direction her life and health were headed and was putting in her best effort to change it.

The problem was she'd done this before and was saddled with the weight of past defeats. She wasn't sure where to focus her efforts and didn't know who she could trust to lead her to the results she desired. She felt overwhelmed in a sea of endless choices, uncertain of where to turn or what to believe.

She'd bought into the lie that diet and exercise were the complete solution to getting healthy again. It felt like a lonely, uphill battle every day.

When she finally saw the whole picture of what it REALLY takes to be healthy AND how easy it can be, a weight came off of her shoulders. She found hope where she had none. A wave of excitement rushed over her as she caught sight of a new vision where she could have the health and energy she had dreamed of for so long.

Because you're reading this book, it's clear you want to be healthy. That's a great start. Everyone wants to be healthy. As you get older, you don't want to end up like so many of your friends and family who are old, broken down, can't live in their own house, and have long since given up the things they love. They've accepted being able to do less and less and convinced themselves that's all that they want to do.

You and I know that's just not true.

You want to be happy and vibrant your whole life, and live to a good, old age so you can experience everything you care about in this world. You want to be able to have fun with your spouse or your kids. You want to be able to do the things that you love. You don't want to have to give them up because your body isn't well.

It doesn't have to be like that. You don't have to be on the sidelines. You can get back in the game! You've only got one life! Live it boldly.

If I asked if you want to be healthy, you'd say "of course!" However, when you look around, are most people healthy? Unfortunately, the answer is no. There's a big disconnect between what they say they want and what they actually have, and you feel it.

You've accepted headaches because you haven't seen anything that worked over the long term. You've accepted taking pills as just part of your life now because no one's shown you how simple it can be to get better naturally. You've accepted the injuries or pains you're dealing with. Don't buy into the lie that this is now part of your life just because no one's been able to show you they can help.

Why this disconnect? Where does it come from? There's a number of reasons, and often it's not your fault. You want to be healthy, but the disappointments from your past can get in the way of doing what you know you need to do to move on.

1. The right information and steps – Maybe you've had these problems for so long that it's very difficult for you to ever see them changing. The habits that you've formed have been there for so long that you don't see how you can do things any other way. You think you're the old dog that can't learn a new trick. Maybe you've been disappointed by diets and products in the past so when you read these words, you think of all the other books and experts that have let you down before.

As a result, your hopes are crushed and you don't see how things can ever change. You're like the young elephant tied to a stake that learns over time that there's no use in trying to uproot it.

The truth is, you can.

That's the reason why starting with your mindset is THE MOST IMPORTANT FIRST STEP. You need to see the reality of how powerful your body really is. When you tap into that and start to convince yourself of a new reality, you find power and strength that you never knew before. Why? Because when you start to see yourself as a healthy person, you look at what you're doing and see that it doesn't match your identity.

"If I'm a healthy person, then the way I've been living doesn't match. There's a disconnect. If I truly believe I'm a healthy person, then my actions must change."

That's what makes it so much easier. You start to believe in yourself more when you find a new identity in yourself.

2. Cut through the clutter – We have too much information. We used to live in a world where it was difficult to understand exactly what it takes to stay healthy. There was a lack of information about what your body really needs. It was easy to be ignorant about what it really takes to stay healthy. As an example, it wasn't too long ago that trans fats weren't that big a deal, artificial sweeteners were billed as healthy, and people ate margarine, thinking it was the smart thing to do.

I don't think that's the case anymore.

With the internet, you have all the information you could possibly want about how to stay healthy. There are more diets, studies, and advice than you know what to do with. All the information you have access to becomes too much for one person to make sense of. As a result, you're paralyzed by all the options.

What you need now is not more information but more FOCUS. Imagine if you had a GUIDE and a COACH to help you wade through that slew of information and find the solid rocks that you can base your life on? It would take away the confusion and doubt, and replace it with more certainty and focus. Timeless principles are what you need. You need principles that are time-tested and proven, not in a laboratory, but by people actually living their life.

That's why we focused on the Blue Zones. They're the people who most often live into their nineties and hundreds and do so with energy, independence, and purpose. You're more likely to get better results mimicking what they're doing to stay healthy than from some scientist in a lab coat who's out of shape by the time he or she is forty.

3. Custom-tailored to you – Your plan needs to be personalized. You need something that's tailor-made just for you and your situation. Your stresses. Your challenges. Your body. What's the next right step for you?

Why is this important? It's important because your life is unique. You're busy. You have a family. You have a business. You have a career to focus on. Your responsibilities are unique. You have all kinds of other priorities. Maybe you're taking care of aging parents AND taking care of kids. You don't have a lot of time to be messing around trying things that don't work. You need a personalized plan. You need the right principles made applicable for you. This way you have the focus and the clarity to be very specific with where you put your time, your energy, and your money.

4. Accountability and Follow-up – You need someone to keep you accountable. The people you choose to be your guides and your healthcare providers are supposed to be there to direct you. Their role is to show you the next step and give you advice on how to handle problems as they come up. They need to spend the time to answer your questions so you're fully informed about what you need to do.

You may feel cheated and alone because your healthcare providers have left you hanging. They promised you the moon, and when you really needed their leadership, they either didn't have the time or they didn't know how to meet your needs. As a result, you feel rushed, processed, not listened to, and alone.

These are some of the biggest reasons why you've quit in the past. It's not your fault. Everything's harder when you go alone. You're leaning only on your own strength, and that's where doubt comes in. After a few bad days, it's very easy to stop and question whether what you're doing is actually going to work for you. Follow-up from someone qualified is the key to keeping you on track and courageously moving toward your goals.

5. A cheerleader in your corner – You need someone on your side who's going to give you the certainty that you're moving in the right direction. You need someone to celebrate your victories with you. Those little victories add up to big changes over time. Victories keep you motivated to continue on the path and do the work to get healthy.

Why is this so important? It's important because it's very difficult to stay healthy in this day and age. It's very, very easy to be sick. Society is set up to keep you average. If you want something different, you have to find somebody who's going to celebrate those victories with you and keep you moving forward in the direction you want.

6. A like-minded community – The last factor is finding a community where people are getting healthier and stronger each year instead of sicker. It's always best if that community is local, but it doesn't have to be. We talked about all the different tools that are available to form a connection with people all over the world. The important step is to find people who support you and have the same values so you don't give up and start going with the flow again.

If you want more, you have to seek it out. The world is not going to give it to you. Every system in our society works to keep you average. When you look at the average, it's not very appealing.

Most people aren't at their best. They have low energy. They don't sleep well. They have brain fog. They're taking medication and dealing with disease, especially as they get older. They've long since given up the things they love and they've accepted that. In their mind, they've accepted the limitations placed on them by their body as a normal part of aging. They see it as beyond their control.

If that sounds like garbage to you, then you have to do something different to change it. Get around people who think differently and expect more. Their habits are going to rub off on you.

Your Solution

All of this is exactly what I do. I believe that every one of us is made for an adventure. That includes you! You are made for an adventure. If you're still breathing, there are improvements that can be made, and incredible experiences and memories waiting for you.

You have unimaginable gifts and talents and abilities inside of you that have the power to transform the world and create a life for you that's beyond what you've ever imagined. That's your birthright. That's ingrained in you and it's immovable. It cannot change.

The question is whether you'll do what it takes to tap into it. A huge part of that is making sure you're healthy enough. If you're busy focusing on health challenges or managing pain, you can't live at your highest level. You can't pursue your hobbies to your highest level. You can't play with your kids the way you want to. You can't enjoy your career or business success the way you dreamed when you first started. Travelling or enjoying retirement becomes so much more difficult. You can't fulfill your purpose like you're meant to.

But when your health is strong, you get to enjoy everything you work and dream so hard for. You get it all, and it's easier than you think!

Here's something to set your imagination on fire: The amount of fun, freedom, and ability you have to tap into grows as your health grows.

As you take steps to improve your health and your life, your capacity to handle new opportunities and challenges increases. The issues and jobs that used to take so much out of you will become easier and more fun over time. What used to be difficult and strenuous will become simpler. It's a beautiful thing!

What do you see for your life? What would you like to see? It's yours, and it's time to get it back!

Just like Stephanie, you can have your own set of custom-tailored solutions, hand-crafted just for you. They're designed around your life and your goals, and are there to give you focus and clarity. You'll know what habits and decisions will give you the results you want the quickest.

It's time to stop putting up with living less than your best. It's time to stop trusting half-way solutions based on fads or weak science. You and your family deserve better than that. You deserve to stay strong and healthy your whole life. I'll show you how to start building that so there's no confusion.

Get Your Own Custom Tailored Plan

If you've read through this book and thought, "This all sounds great, but I'm going to need some help," that's where I come in. Having someone with the knowledge base to guide you makes all the difference between success and struggle.

Having worked in a large multidisciplinary clinic with medical doctors, chiropractors, and massage therapists, I've seen what's done well and what's done poorly in terms of taking care of people. My clinic is set up with a slower pace so you can get real answers when you need them. All your recommendations are custom tailored for your situation and your goals.

This gives you the certainty of knowing that you're putting your time, energy, and money into something that's the next right step for you. I'll help you make sense of the glut of information out there and find the areas to focus on. It's about timeless, unchanging, reliable principles, not trendy fads.

When you meet with me, I 100% guarantee that you will leave with a plan, custom tailored just for you, with clearly defined short-term steps and long-term goals. You will have a plan and a coach. What more do you really need? All you need to bring is your willingness to dream bigger, take positive steps, and stay accountable. Isn't that exciting?!

It's about personalized service and being your cheerleader. It's about being part of a community that's giving you exactly what you need to stay healthy. It's about connecting you to like-minded people and fantastic opportunities to take your health to the next level. It's for people who want to kick ass and never grow old.

I will connect you to the proven nutritional advice. I will teach you how to create a chemical-free home. I will teach you the most effective exercises. I will teach you about nerve supply and how to create strong, robust health. I will teach you about forging a winning mindset. On top of that, I'll show you how to build it into your life without sacrificing your other priorities or responsibilities!

And we'll make it fun!

When the dust settles, you can be a health leader among your family and friends. They'll look at your life and want what you have. You'll feel great in your body and feel great about your choices. You'll feel powerful. You'll feel unstoppable. I'll lead you there!

TO SEE WHAT YOU CAN EXPECT FROM YOUR FIRST
SESSION WITH ME, AND TO GET STARTED WITH YOUR
OWN CUSTOM TAILORED SOLUTION,
SCAN THE QR CODE BELOW
OR GO TO

WWW.ITSNOTYOURFAULTYOUVEBEENLIEDTO.COM/
BOOK-BONUSES

Chapter 7
Here's Where it Gets
Even More Exciting!!!

"Small deeds done are better than big deeds planned."

– Peter Marshall

So where do you go from here?

You know the system is stacked against you. You've been sold a lie and told to put your trust in a way of thinking that's not delivering the kind of health you know you should have. However, it's still your body, so ultimately it's up to you to decide what kind of health you create for yourself and your family. The good news is, you have everything you need.

Remember the intro to this book? You need the right information and the right support. You are now on the path to the right information. You also have the right support in me. You've seen how important it is to take your health into your hands. More importantly, you've seen how simple it can be. When you cut out the clutter, the enduring principles remain, and they are ROCK SOLID.

Start Small but Start Quickly

These principles have worked for thousands of years across cultures. Be confident in them. Change only a few things at a time. Do them consistently before making another new change. Make it easy to win. The more consistent you are with a few things, the more momentum you'll have. That momentum will lead to more changes. Over time, you'll craft the kind of life and health you want.

Just like Stephanie, we are starting a journey together. Nothing worthwhile happens overnight without work. However, the more you connect to your new identity, the work we do will become a joy as you uncover more of your true nature.

Instead of a constant fight against deeply entrenched habits, I'll help you more easily walk into habits that will reveal the vibrant person you were always meant to be.

It's been a beautiful thing to watch as the blinders and lies fall away from my clients' eyes. Too often you've accepted far less and then convinced yourself that the box you created for yourself is all you need.

I invite you to look up. Look around you. See the limitations that your friends and family place on themselves every day, and then reject those limits. You're more powerful than you realize. Your goals are within your reach. Change your mind and all else follows from there.

Remember that everything begins in your mind first. You see the results you want before they ever become a reality. Connect to the results, and connect to them often. Even if you think you're lying to yourself in the beginning, know that changes are coming. Envision what you want and declare "THIS IS WHO I AM!" From there, your habits and beliefs will start to change and all the other steps will be so much easier for you.

You are not unhealthy. You've just made many unhealthy choices up to this point.

You've trusted a system that is great at keeping you alive but unhealthy. Look for the people who have what you want.

Build Over Time

Remember to be gracious with yourself. If you've never realized how powerful these simple changes can be, or you've been inconsistent in the past, that's ok. Celebrate each small victory and build over time. Master one principle before you move on to the next.

In my life, I've failed many times. MANY times! I've kicked myself when I was down, and I was my own harshest critic. I felt I was weak for giving in to temptations, and a hypocrite for not always following my own advice. However, the best thing I've ever done was to lay a foundation of how I saw myself. I deliberately carved time out of my day to imagine the feeling of achieving the goal I was striving for. And when I fell, I was grateful for taking time beforehand to build relationships with people who would lift me up, dust me off, and encourage me to keep going.

This is why my brother contributed in the beginning of this book. He was a huge cheerleader for me through the years, and brought me back into line with the goals I set.

Find great people around you who want you to succeed, then stick with them. Together you'll be stronger and achieve more.

Your Action Plan

Below is a short list of the areas we will talk about together when you take the first step to work with me in creating the life you want:

1. First, determine what you want.
   a. Forget what you think is realistic; define your dream. Make it real. Write it down. Connect to it daily.

2. Define your reality.

    a. You can't create the life you want without knowing where you are now. Be honest with yourself, even if it hurts. The good news is that the struggles you're facing have been overcome by others before you. They've been overcome before, which means you can overcome them too.

3. Know your roadblocks.

    a. Identify where you've struggled in the past and how you can overcome them.

    b. Is it difficult to find time to make healthy meals? How can you have it ready ahead of time?

    c. Is it painful for you to exercise? What can you do RIGHT NOW that you can improve on as you get better?

    d. Do you emotionally eat? How can you connect to your unique and beautiful gifts and abilities that will remind you of your worth and value?

    e. Have two solutions ready for each roadblock you identify. This way you're prepared beforehand when temptation inevitably comes.

4. Find the right people with the right information.

    a. Find out how they build healthy habits into their lifestyle. Right now, you have all the keys you need to see a MASSIVE transformation in your body and to do in a sustainable way.

5. Get up when you fall down.

    a. Connect to your true identity and recognize that you are not your illness, and you are not your mistakes. Get back up and courageously step forward again.

The resources in this book are for you. Use them, and use them often. Just like any new skill, you'll have to connect to it again and again. In fact, I encourage you to **read this book once a week for the first month.**

Taking in this information on a consistent basis will begin to change your identity and habits in a powerful and lasting way.

These principles have been tested by life, and by people who have lived long, happy, healthy lives, full of purpose, significance, joy, and independence. They've been able to fully experience this beautiful world and the wonderful people in it. They've kept a smile on their face and joy in their heart.

You can have it too.

Now is the time for courage. Let go of the past. Look to the future. Define your dream and take the first step forward. This is in your hands now. You have all the tools you need. You don't have to live like most people; tired, sick, and in pain. You were made for more, and the exciting part is you have everything you need right now. There's nothing stopping you from creating the life you know you were always meant to live.

Reject the lies. Connect to these timeless principles. It's time to LIVE YOUR BEST LIFE NOW. I am here for YOU. Click the links below and let's get started.

FOR ALL OF THE BONUSES FROM THE BOOK,
AND TO GET STARTED WITH YOUR OWN CUSTOM
TAILORED SOLUTION, EMAIL ME AT
INFO@ELEVATIONCHIROPRACTIC.CA
SCAN THE QR CODE BELOW
OR GO TO

WWW.ITSNOTYOURFAULTYOUVEBEENLIEDTO.COM/
BOOK-BONUSES

References

1. Adams KM, Kohlmeier M, Zeisel SH. Nutrition education in U.S. medical schools: latest update of a national survey. Acad Med. 2010 Sep;85(9):1537-42.

2. Starfield B. Is US Health Really the Best in the World?. JAMA. 2000;284(4):483-485.

3. http://www.cdc.gov/chronicdisease/stats/. August 3, 2015

4. Moore, David S. (2015). The Developing Genome: An Introduction to Behavioral Epigenetics (1st ed.). Oxford University Press. ISBN 978-0199922345.

5. http://www.breastcancerdeadline2020.org/breast-cancer-information/myths-and-truths/myth-13-everyone-with-BCRA1-or-2-gets-bc.html. October 2015.

6. Riggs AD, Russo VEA, Martienssen RA (1996). Epigenetic mechanisms of gene regulation. Plainview, N.Y.: Cold Spring Harbor Laboratory Press. ISBN 0-87969-490-4

7. Buettner, D. (2012). The Blue Zones: 9 lessons for living longer from the people who've lived the longest.

8. Freedhoff, Dr. Yoni. Canada's Food Guide is broken – and no one wants to fix it. Globe and Mail. April 16, 2015.

9. Brasco, Joseph. Low Grain and Carbohydrate Diets Treat Hypoglycemia, Heart Disease, Diabetes, Cancer and Nearly ALL Chronic Illness. http://www.mercola.com/article/carbohydrates/scientific_evidence_low_grains.htm. October 8, 2015.

10. http://www.webmd.com/arthritis/about-inflammation. Oct 8, 2015.

11. Marquis, David M. How Inflammation Affects Every Aspect of Your Health. http://articles.mercola.com/sites/articles/archive/2013/03/07/inflammation-triggers-disease-symptoms.aspx. March 7, 2013.

12. Casey, John. Diet Sabotage: How Much Sugar Are You Eating? http://www.medicinenet.com/script/main/art.asp?articlekey=56589

13. WebMD. High Blood Sugar, Diabetes, and Your Body. Reviewed by Michael Dansinger, MD. Sept 3, 2014.

14. Warburg, O. On the origin of cancer cells. Science 1956 Feb;123:309-14

15. Silberstein, Susan. 5 Reasons Sugar and Cancer Are Best Friends. www.beatcancer.org.

16. Kaaks R, Energy balance and cancer: the role of insulin and insulin-like growth factor-1. Proc Nutr Soc 2001 Feb;60(1):91-106

17. Mercola, Joseph. Alzheimer's – A Disease Fed By Sugar. www.drmercola.com. August 13, 2015

18. Wells, S. D. U.S. treating meat with ammonia, bleach and antibiotics to kill the '24-hour sickness'. www.naturalnews.com. March 29, 2014.

19. Alenda, Andrea. Somatosensation. http://www.fastbleep.com/biology-notes/39/145/911. Oct 9, 2015

20. National Space Biomedical Research Institute. http://www.nsbri.org/DISCOVERIES-FOR-SPACE-and-EARTH/The-Body-in-Space/. Oct 9, 2015.

21. Griffin, R. Morgan. Your Kid's Brain on Exercise. www.webmd.com. Reviewed By Hansa D. Bhargava, MD. Oct 9, 2015.

22. Fightforkids.org. Facts and Statistics. www.fightforkids.org. Oct 9, 2015.

23. Blumenthal, James A. Effects of Exercise Training on Older Patients with Major Depression. Arch Intern Med. 1999;159(19):2349-2356.

24. Schmidt, Wilfred Daniel (1992). The effects of aerobic and anaerobic exercise on resting metabolic rate, thermic effect of a meal, and excess post exercise oxygen consumption. Purdue University.

25. Baylor LS1, Hackney AC. Resting thyroid and leptin hormone changes in women following intense, prolonged exercise training. Eur J Appl Physiol. 2003 Jan;88(4-5):480-4. Epub 2002 Nov 22.

26. Wescott, T. et al. A meta-analysis of the past 25 years of weight loss research using diet, exercise or diet plus exercise intervention. International Journal of Obesity. 1997. 21. 941-947.

27. Mercola, Joseph. Peak Fitness: This Simple Trick Stops Aging in its Tracks. www.drmercola.com. Oct 9, 2015.

28. Halden, Rolf U. Plastics and Health Risks. Annual Review of Public Health. Vol. 31: 179-194

29. Mytilineou C1, Kramer BC, Yabut JA. Glutathione depletion and oxidative stress. Parkinsonism Relat Disord. 2002 Sep;8(6):385-7.

30. Droge, Wulf, Raoul Breitkreutz. Glutathione and Immune Function. Proceedings of the Nutrition Society (2000), 59, 595–600

31. Gutman, Jimmy. "Therapeutic Potential of Glutathione Augmentation in Cancer Patients Receiving Chemotherapy or Radiotherapy". Journal of Nutritional Oncology, November 15, 2016, Volume 1, Number 1. 40-44

32. Kandel ER, Schwartz JH, Jessel TM, eds. (2000). "Ch. 2: Nerve cells and behavior". Principles of Neural Science. McGraw-Hill Professional. ISBN 978-0-8385-7701-1.

33. Videman, T. Experimental models of osteoarthritis: the role of immobilization. Clinical Biomechanics. 1987. issue 2:223-229

34. Yochum, Terry R , and Lindsay J. Rowe. Essentials of Skeletal Radiology 2nd ed. 2 vols. Ed. John P. Butler. Baltimore: Willaims and Wilkins, 1996

35. Reid, J.D, "Effects of Flexion-Extension Movements of the Head and Spine upon the Spinal Cord and Nerve Roots", J. Neurology Neurosurgery and Psychiatry, 1960, 23: 214-221

36. Rhodes, Walter R. The Official History of Chiropractic in Texas. Texas Chiropractic Association, 1978.

37. Pettman E. A History of Manipulative Therapy. The Journal of Manual & Manipulative Therapy. 2007;15(3):165-174.

38. Winsor, H. Sympathetic segmental disturbances – II. The evidences of the association, in dissected cadavers, of visceral disease with vertebral deformities of the same sympathetic segments, The Medical Times, November 1921, pp./ 267-271.

www.ingramcontent.com/pod-product-compliance
Lightning Source LLC
Chambersburg PA
CBHW071156280526
45787CB00002B/523